MY FIGHT FOR SANITY

by Judith Kruger

This is a true story. It is a dramatic story. It spotlights, in frank and intimate impressions, what it is like to be mentally ill. Written in gripping, personal style, it describes a woman's mental breakdown following the birth of her child.

With utter frankness – the words taken right out of her diary written day by day in the mental hospital – the author describes her daily life as a mental patient, the impossible yet somehow endurable days and nights of ward routine, her terror preceding the electric shock treatments.

Here, in the bright light of truth, the reader sees how thin is the tightrope between sickness and sanity, and is immediately drawn into this woman's torment and flight from reality as she attempts to blot out with self-destruction her fear of what is happening to her. You will be shocked and stunned by her candid revelations.

It was her doctor who suggested that she write about her experiences as her depression and fears passed away and she began to gain strength and spontaneity in her feelings again, and here is the result of her efforts.

18s.
net

MY FIGHT FOR SANITY

MY FIGHT FOR SANITY

This is a true story. It is a dramatic story. It spotlights, in frank and intimate impressions, what it is like to be mentally ill. Written in gripping, personal style, it describes a woman's mental breakdown following the birth of her child.

With utter frankness—the words taken right out of her diary written day by day in the mental hospital— the author describes her daily life as a mental patient, the impossible yet somehow endurable days and nights of ward routine, her terror preceding the electric shock treatments.

Here, in the bright light of truth, the reader sees how thin is the tightrope between sickness and sanity, and is immediately drawn into this woman's torment and flight from reality as she attempts to blot out with self-destruction her fear of what is happening to her.

It was her doctor who suggested that she should write about her experiences as her depression and fears passed away and she began to gain strength and spontaneity in her feelings again, and here is the result of her efforts.

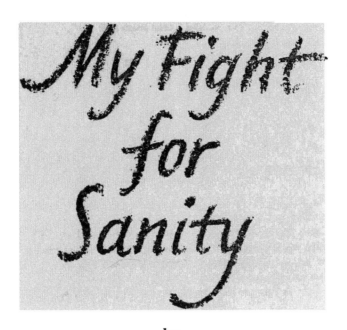

My Fight for Sanity

by

JUDITH KRUGER

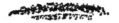

LONDON

HAMMOND, HAMMOND

AND COMPANY

FOREWORD

This is the story of a mental breakdown.

It is my story, and my fight, with the help of psychotherapy, to regain mental health.

I began this chronicle at the suggestion of my doctor, after I had been in treatment for a few months. When he said to me, 'Why don't you write about your experience?' I recoiled. Recent events were still too fresh and too full of pain, and my confidence in past abilities was shattered. But, as the weeks passed, I grew well enough to face my self-inflicted trial and by so doing moved a little closer to emotional maturity.

But this is not my only reason for writing.

Rarely are we interested in the difficulties of others until we ourselves are catapulted into personal tragedy. Since my illness, I have found a bond with people like me, and, through research from professional and lay articles, a deeper understanding of the forces that govern our actions and determine our ability to meet life or flee from it into a world of darkness.

My story is a true one. All events are as they actually happened. But, in order to protect their identities, I have used fictitious names for members of my family and all persons and places directly involved. Beyond this, no attempt at fictionization has been made.

It is not a pretty story. There is no happy ending . . . only a long beginning.

The Author

No one can develop in a vacuum.

The adult personality is a product of two determining forces—hereditary characteristics and emotional environment. The seed of self must grow in soil, a soil which can nurture or stunt.

Despite economic security and an average middle-class background, my seed of development had unhealthy roots. But they were hidden and deep, and, until the birth of my child, I had functioned adequately with no signs of the emotional storm that was to come.

I met my husband shortly after I was graduated from a New York City college. He had just been released from the Navy and was ready to complete his undergraduate studies at a southern university. We were married two years later when he received his degree and I moved South with him. He spent one more year in study for his Master's degree and then received an acceptance to medical school.

I used the long hours when he was studying to write short stories and to write and direct amateur musical comedies for a group of university students. Then I became active in a local theatre group. Soon acting became a source of supreme satisfaction. I released my excess energy in comic roles and found great pleasure in having people watch and laugh and clap their hands for me.

My letters home were accompanied by news clippings of productions in which I had performed, and my family and friends were properly awed at my ability to hold a job, keep house, and participate in outside activities.

On the surface, it was a neat package of a life. I was active, efficient, and very productive, and envisaged the later years when I would be the wife of a professional man and mother to at least three children. Our home would be beautiful and well organized, and I would be on the programme committees of half a dozen women's clubs. And yet there were occasional flurries and ripplings of anxiety that disturbed me. I was very serious and intent about all household chores. I tackled every task with tension, whether it was cooking, shopping, getting clothes back from the cleaners on time, or whatever. And I was frightened of change—a new job, a trip, moving to a new apartment—anything.

When my husband was in his junior year at medical school, we talked of having a child. We both wanted children, but each in a different way. To my husband, a baby would be a natural extension of himself whose growth would enrich him emotionally and enhance our marriage. I too wanted a baby, but my hunger was like that of a child who covets another's lollipop or toy.

Before I met my husband, I envied my girl friends their dates. I stared at wedding rings on the hands of women in the subways. When I found Jay and marriage, I was temporarily satisfied, but then I started to hunger again, this time for whatever was next on the list of 'things' to have in life—a baby.

But I didn't attain my desire easily. My menstrual cycles were irregular. And, as time passed, I became so obsessed with the yearning to conceive that I could not express it to my husband. Finally I went to a gynæcologist, who assured me that he did not consider me a sterility case. He gave me a prescription and told me to check my temperature each morning. I faithfully took the pills and every day I counted and recounted each rise and fall in the temperature curve.

I never intimated to family or friends how desperately I was trying to have a baby, for I knew that their questions would only add to my obsession. And in all of her letters my mother never prodded me or hinted, 'Well, aren't you two thinking of a child yet? You've been married four years.' Or, as many mothers do, 'When will you give us a grandchild?'

She didn't have to ask. I felt it inside—a wrenching desire to see them as grandparents, to give them the pleasure of my child. It was almost as if my baby would be a gift to them, a repayment, a sure sign of appreciation. Appreciation for what?—I didn't know.

That September I enjoyed a suspicion that I was pregnant. I

had missed a period. The temperature curve stayed up. My husband and I shared delicious moments of anticipation.

Finally I called my gynæcologist. He was away on holiday and another doctor was in his office. He told me to bring a urine specimen which he would give to the laboratory for the 'frog test'.

I waited the prescribed number of days, then nervously dialled him from my office. He wasn't in, so I left my business number. Unfortunately, I was away from my desk when he called, and the girl who took the message gave me the wrong telephone listing. It was like a comedy of errors, but finally I reached him that evening at his home. My voice betrayed my anxiety.

'Doctor,' I stammered, 'what was the result?'

'Oh, Mrs. Kruger,' he said, his voice young and friendly, 'one of the frogs died.'

'Died?' I echoed.

'Yes. It happens very often. That's why they use two frogs for the test.'

'Well, what about the other one?'

'The results were inconclusive. You'll have to bring another specimen. I hope you don't mind?'

'Oh, no. Of course not! I'll bring it tomorrow.'

I hung up, a little disappointed. Then, with exaggerated humour, I made a joke of it.

'Darling,' I said, 'one frog died and the other wouldn't commit himself. Poor dead frog. I wonder what did him in? It must have been the soda pop and hot dogs at the office party yesterday.'

We laughed and intoned a requiem for the recently deceased.

The second test left nothing in doubt. It was positive. I was pregnant! I was going to have a baby! And yet, I still lied to family, friends, and business associates. I acted very naïve and led them to believe that the pregnancy wasn't planned. 'A sort of accident', I murmured. Somehow I could not say openly, comfortably, 'I'm pregnant', without excuses and hemming and hawing.

The months flew by and I enjoyed good health, working until three weeks before the baby was born.

We had frequent talks about moving to Philadelphia soon after the baby's birth in order that Jay might be ready for his internship in a Philadelphia hospital. All the details were worked out. My mother would come down and stay with me while Jay travelled by car to Philly to a sublet apartment. Then we would follow by train. I visualized the entire procedure, down to the last bottle of milk in the refrigerator, the dress I would wear on the train, and where to buy disposable nappies. And I alternated between nervous anticipation and cocky confidence.

'Everything'll be all right', I told myself. 'I'll handle it.'

But there were vague stirrings of fear. I tried to push them away by poring over Doctor Spock's book on baby care, underlining and memorizing all the important chapters. I tackled the book like a college text, to make sure I would get straight 'A's' on all the facts I'd been cramming.

Our son, Gary Edward, was born on the third of June. He weighed six pounds, three ounces. Jay saw him a few minutes after delivery. He wasn't crying at all—his dark brown eyes were wide open and staring into space.

I can't remember when they brought him to me for the first time, how he looked lying next to me in the bed, the feeling I had when I nursed him, or the ride home in the car, yet I do remember taking home one of the hospital cot pads. I did it deliberately. I told myself that they had so many and that it was half-worn anyway, and that maybe I didn't have enough at home. I stole it because I was always afraid to use up my own things. When I was acting with the theatre group, I bought paper tissues for use in make-up but I hoarded them and instead used the tissues belonging to other members of the cast. Tissues and strings and shoelaces and cot pads: inexpensive things, unimportant to everyone but me.

Gary cried almost constantly the first night we came home and I was very worried, but not about him. Our apartment was sectioned off from the landlady's quarters and I was terribly upset about waking her and how nice she was and wasn't it a shame how we were disturbing her.

My mother arrived from New York at six the next morning. It had been an exciting week for her. First had come our

telegram announcing Gary's birth, then she had gone to up-
state New York to attend my brother's college graduation,
and now she had taken an aeroplane trip to see her first grandchild.

She came in flushed and happy and stared in wonderment at
the baby, who was finally asleep in his bassinet. I was very glad
to see her, more than I would admit to myself.

'How was the trip, Mom? Were you airsick?'

'Oh, no. I had a good sleep. Look at that darling! I can't
believe it!'

'How's Dad? And Harold? How was the graduation?'

'Fine. Wonderful. He gave us a nice time. He got me a
corsage for the graduation. How are *you*, how was the labour?
Was the baby a good boy last night?'

'Well, he cried a lot. Take off your hat, Mom. Give me the
suitcase.'

'Are you all right? You feel well?'

'Yes. Nervous, you know? I mean, I don't sleep well. Jay got
me some sedatives from the doctor——'

'Oh, we're all nervous the first few weeks. Are you breast-
feeding? What kind of formula? Do you . . .?'

'Want some coffee, Mom? Did you eat? How's Dad?'

'Fine.' She moved to the bassinet again. 'I just can't believe
he's here. It's all like a dream . . . the telegram . . .'

'He's here, all right', I said.

And my voice echoed in my ears, *Here . . . he's here . . . he's
here . . . and I'm scared, scared, scared!*

Mother slept in a room at the back of the house which was
vacant. She was with me constantly and we fluttered and
hovered over the baby. At first, she was afraid to hold him. But
I wasn't. I handled him adequately, even cutting his fingernails. I attended nicely to his physical needs. But I couldn't
sleep. I needed more and more sedation.

The next week, Jay began to study for the State Board
Medical exams. It was hard for him to concentrate in the small
apartment with the new baby. The exams lasted three days,
and he was away most of that time. I didn't miss him—I was
consumed in mounting tension. It was like a cloud round me, a

choking fog. I had no inkling of what was wrong. I only knew that I was more nervous than I had ever been in my life.

The apartment looked so different, so disorganized—the dresser piled with clean nappies, the sterilizing equipment in the sink, baby things covering desks and chairs, and open cartons all round waiting for final packing.

On June 16th, Jay left for the car trip to Philadelphia. He had arranged for a sublet apartment there through contact with his internship hospital. The back seat and the boot of the car were filled with household articles—dishes, radios, brooms, typewriter, irons, cutlery, tools, and balanced on top of everything our ironing board. Jay looked like a travelling salesman who lugs the warehouse with him.

I stood near the kerb, watching the car chug down the street, and felt a new wave of fear rise in me. Then I rushed back into the house to count my sleeping pills.

Five days later, my mother and I were ready to leave, with reservations for a compartment on the train to Philadelphia. On previous trips to New York I had travelled by coach. Now I looked forward to the relative luxury of a compartment. As it turned out, though, the trip was a fiasco. Everything went wrong, except the direction of the train. It, at least, was on the right track, heading north.

Things started satisfactorily enough. Gary was an angel. He slept soundly when the taxicab driver lifted his bassinet into the cab. Our landlady stood on the steps of the house waving us a fond farewell. We could have said our good-byes ten times over while the patient driver made six other trips from house to cab bearing our luggage and cartons.

At the railway station lights were blazing. Baggage trucks rumbled up and down the stone corridors and the loud-speakers were blaring. But all the hubbub served merely to keep Gary asleep.

The station porter lifted the bassinet up into the train, and my mother and I followed him down the corridor to our little home away from home. Little was right! A compartment is meant for two persons travelling light. Not for two plus a baby plus a bassinet plus nineteen pieces of assorted paraphernalia.

We strew our things about haphazardly. The first thing was

to find our porter to give him the bottles to put in the refrigerator. I was still breast-feeding, but we had prepared a formula as a precaution.

Button, button, where was the porter's button? We looked behind the bed, over the bed, under the bed. I even peered into the toilet compartment, which bore no resemblance to any toilet I'd ever seen since the main article of necessity was nowhere to be seen. We felt up and down the walls like children in the blindfolded game of 'Pin the Tail on the Donkey'. Still no button.

Finally, I stuck my head out of the door and called, 'Yoo, hoo, Porter!' A fat man edged by, eyeing me strangely. I lurched into the corridor and the door slammed shut.

I fumbled for the knob to open it, but no knob. No buttons and now no doorknobs. A letter to the president of the railway was angrily taking shape in my mind, a letter which, had I undertaken it at the end of the trip, would have consumed ten pages, all single-spaced.

'Mother,' I called, 'let me in! I can't find the thing to open the door!'

No answer. Just the rumble of the train.

'Mo-ther! Open up! *Open the door!*'

The fat man edged by again, staring suspiciously. I returned a what-the-hell-are-you-looking-at glare and pounded on the door, trying to shout above the clack of the wheels.

Suddenly a porter appeared.

'Ma'am?'

'Oh, are you our porter?'

'Yes, ma'am. Can I help you?' The poor soul didn't know that this casual inquiry would place him in our bondage for the rest of the trip.

'What's the trouble, ma'am?'

'I can't get in.'

'Is this your compartment?'

'Of course it's my compartment! My mother's in there and we couldn't find your button. We've got bottles to be put on ice and now I'm locked out.'

He looked at me strangely. He probably thought that I was tight and that it wasn't my mother in there but a gentleman

friend and that the bottles to be put on ice were filled with
champagne. He didn't say anything—he just smiled. Porters are
very diplomatic. Then he reached down and clicked a thing-a-
ma-jig by the side of the door. It opened like sesame.

. Mother was sitting in the corner, half-hidden by luggage,
with one hand on the bassinet, rocking to the rhythm of the rails.

I pointed her out to him like a guide on a Cook's tour.

'That's my mother.'

'Yes, ma'am.'

'That's my baby.'

'Yes, ma'am.'

'I've got bottles. Formula bottles. For the baby. Could you
put them in the kitchen refrigerator for us?'

'Well, no, I couldn't do that. But I can get some ice and keep
them cold in a bucket.'

'Oh, fine! Fine. Thank you so much.'

And for the next two days he kept vigil over the bottles. And
Gary never needed them! He slept most of the time and I
breast-fed him when he was awake. So before the train reached
Philadelphia we gulped six ice-cold bottles of formula, more to
save face before the porter than anything else.

When the porter left us that first evening he showed us the
button to press if we wanted him. It was embedded near the
door and painted the same colour as the walls.

Mother and I started shifting things about like longshoremen
unloading cargo. Suddenly the porter was knocking.

'Did you ring?'

'No.'

'The bell rang.'

'No. I'm sorry. We didn't ring.'

Twice in the next two hours the same thing happened again.
He came, unheralded. He was losing patience fast.

'You sure? You real sure you didn't press the button? The
one I showed you?'

'No.'

Then he took in the scene of cramped confusion, pursed his
lips in studied thought, and said, 'Well, maybe with all this
bumpin' 'n' movin' you been doing, you maybe leaned on it
a little.'

'Well!' I said. 'Yeah . . . that could be. You're right. I didn't realize. I mean . . . Hah! That's funny!'

His face was stony. He didn't share the joke.

'Yes, ma'am', he said, tight-lipped.

He closed the door to our suppressed laughter.

Now it was time to bed down for the night. But we had not yet investigated the bathroom facilities. We peered into the dark cavity leading off from the compartment.

'Where are the lights?' Mother asked.

'Oh, goodness!' I exploded. 'More buttons! Be careful, now, the porter may pop in again. Oh, there's a button, Mother. On the wall. I'm going to press it. If a sink or a toilet falls from the ceiling, duck!'

But all was well. After a few moments' hesitation, a fluorescent light came on. The bathroom was very complete and compact, a marvel of the machine age. But it required excellent co-ordination to control with one hand the pressurized tap that either dribbled or gushed, retrieve the latherless soap that slipped from the other hand, and stand out of the way of the swinging door that flapped to and fro with each turn of the train.

The toilet itself was tolerable—it served its purpose. But it took the strength of ten men to press the flush pedal. And the call of nature seemed always to coincide with hour-long train stops.

Outside our windows it was a torrid ninety-two degrees; inside, we were freezing. Torrents of cold air rushed through the air-conditioning vents. With teeth chattering we stuffed wads of paper hankies and underwear up into the grilles, huddled under coats on the couches, too tired to find out how they opened into beds. And somehow the night went by.

Gary woke early. We creaked to our feet. I fed him, changed him, and got his wind up. Now it was time to think of food for ourselves.

We had sandwiches packed in an overnight case which was sitting in the bathroom. But dry food at seven in the morning is unappetizing. Juice and plenty of coffee was what we needed.

I eased out of the compartment and shuffled through the cars to the dining-car. I found a seat alone since I was in no mood to make chit-chat with a stranger. I tried to look out at the countryside growing bright with the sun. But I couldn't enjoy the view. Somehow it hurt to look at the world around me. I was too tight and too tense inside. Each time I thought of my baby I had to turn my head from the window.

I gulped the coffee and stumbled back. The narrowness of the corridors and the noise of the train seemed to accentuate my nervousness.

Mother had planned to go for breakfast as soon as I returned. But Gary chose this moment for his first crying spell of the trip, and she didn't have a chance to leave until a full hour later. And we were so busy we didn't realize that the train had stopped, shuffled, chugged, and wrenched itself up and back in station sidings for almost twenty minutes.

'Look, Mom. It's almost nine o'clock. Go get some breakfast or the dining-car'll be closed.'

'All right.' She was by the door.

'It's just two cars up that way.' I pointed forward. 'You can't miss it.'

But she did. She missed it by at least fifteen cars. She came back half an hour later, sat down, and waved her hand vaguely.

'What's the matter, Mom?'

'I didn't want coffee, anyway.'

She sat there, puffing.

'For heaven's sake, what happened? You look exhausted.'

'I just couldn't find it.'

'Find what?'

'The car. The dining-car. It's not there.'

'What do you mean, "not there"?'

'Just what I said. Not there.' She was getting her breath back. 'I started front. You said two cars up, remember? Well, I went up front. I opened and closed about thirty doors. I kept going and going. I must have been right up to the locomotive.'

'There's no locomotive on this train. It's a diesel.'

'Diesel, schmiesel—I was almost up riding with the engineer. Then I saw it. A tiny card stuck in a door. It said, "Dining-Car Moved to Rear".'

'So did you go?'

'Where?'

'Back to the rear?'

'No. No, I didn't. I came back here. I'm tired. Go into the bathroom and get me a cheese sandwich and an orange, please.'

I was fumbling with the overnight case stuffed with fruit and sandwiches when she called out, 'I wonder how they did it.'

'Did what?'

'Moved a whole big car like that.'

It gave her food for thought for the rest of the trip.

The apartment we occupied in Philadelphia for a few weeks was sublet from a fourth-year medical student who was away for the summer with his wife and baby. We had never met them, and my immediate reaction on seeing the neighbourhood was one of panic. I couldn't understand how his wife managed. The house was in a hotel-business district and shopping stores were a good distance away. I tramped for blocks under the shadow of the Market Street elevated, clutching my chicken-scratching shopping lists. And I wandered through the aisles of strange stores, cans and boxes falling from my hands. I forgot so many things and would burst into tears when I came home.

Nothing looked right to me. The place was so disorganized. And when my father and brother made their first visit to us, the sight of their faces upset me.

And nothing worked right. The washing machine was a wringer-type and the wringer was a mangler. It chewed up a sheet and a pillowcase before we gave them both up as a bad job and washed clothes in the laundry tubs.

Then there was the refrigerator, a strictly ante-bellum model. The couple had left detailed instructions as to which service company to call in case anything went wrong. Their precautions must have been based on bitter experience, for the machine had malevolence in every cold coil. It defrosted when it felt like it. And when it wanted to work it would start up in the middle of the night, whirring and humming like a turbine.

One afternoon it seemed to give up the ghost. It completely defrosted and dripped water all over the floor. The serviceman we called tinkered with it for over an hour, set the controls, and told us to watch it.

2

'Should frost up in an hour or so', he said, as he picked up his tools.

I followed him to the door. 'Will it be all right?' I asked. 'What's the matter with it? We have so much stuff in there——'

He turned with a what-does-she-want-a-course-in-refrigeration look. 'Look, lady, it's old. You wouldn't work so good if you was old, would you?'

I had no sympathy for the age of the machine. I hated it, as I did everything mechanical that didn't perform perfectly. I sat down next to Jay on the step leading to the pantry and smoked endless cigarettes waiting for the crisis to pass and life to show in the ailing monster. Slowly, it developed frost, but it relapsed the next day and Jay had to drive out to the service company to bring back the man with replacement parts.

I moved thickly through the days. Panic was rising and spreading like a slow paralysis. Sedatives had less and less effect.

On July 1st Jay began his internship in the hospital, with a heavy schedule of work and night duty. On his evenings off he looked for an apartment for us. I knew he was worried about me, for I heard him asking questions of my mother when he came home. I saw him watching me covertly. I wanted to smile for him, to be fresh and crisp when he walked in the door, to lie in bed with him at night. But it was impossible. I was different. I was a strange somebody who couldn't see or feel or move beyond a growing wall of fear.

He came home one evening to find me sitting dejectedly on the edge of the bed. He walked over to me.

'Judith, take this.'

'What is it?' I said, dully. He had a small white pill in his open hand.

'It's medicine to stop the flow of milk in your breasts. Sweetie, you have to get away for a little while. I know a doctor who can admit you to a hospital here in Philly.'

I looked at his face. His eyes were large with worry.

'No. I don't want to.' I thought that to stop breast-feeding would do harm to my child and to me. It would destroy the last shred of reality to which I clung so tenaciously—the illusion that I was all right but just very, very nervous. I tried to explain this

to him, but it was too much of an effort to talk. Instead, I
shook my head from side to side.

'Why won't you take the pill, sweetie?'

'Don't want to go to the hospital.'

'It's just for a short time.' He was bending down now,
squatting on his heels in front of me. 'It'll be good for you.
You'll get a rest. You need a rest, Judy. Don't worry about
Gary. He'll be fine. Now take this.'

I heard his words as if from far away. I stared at the pill.

'Take it, please.'

'What will they do? Put a binder on? Will it hurt?'

'Your breasts will feel sore and full for a day or so. That's all.
Then the milk will stop flowing and you'll be just as you were
before.'

*As before . . . What was before? Was it ever different from this?
This fear. This terror.*

'Take it!' His hand was under my chin now. 'I'm telling you
to take it!'

My arm felt like lead as I lifted it, took the pill, and swallowed it. . . .

Jay's acquaintance, Doctor Downey, had me admitted to the
hospital as a medical case with possible thyroid dysfunction. I
was placed in a large, sunny room with three other patients, but
I spent little time in conversation. I drew the curtain round my
bed and tried to shut out the murmur of their voices. My breasts
were sore and full and quite painful. The nurses gave me medicine for two days and wrapped a binder round me to constrict
the breasts. I was very hot and very uncomfortable.

Most of the ambulatory patients sought relief from the heat on
the patio roof of the hospital, reserved for private and semi-
private patients. There was a flagstone walk, rockers, chaise-
longues, with a fine view of the city to enjoy.

The very first time I went up to the roof I found myself
irresistibly drawn to the railing, and I stood there desperately
clutching the ironwork and staring over the edge. Then I tried
to relax in a chaise-longue, forcing myself to lie back, to rest,
to enjoy the cool breeze. But my hands gripped the arms until
the knuckles went white.

I rushed back to the lift and down to my room. I had to take a bath. A cool bath. Clean myself. I was hot and dirty. Very dirty. I wrung out the washcloth when I was finished and laid it on the edge of the tub. But something made me pick it up again, hide it under my nightgown, and stuff it into my suitcase. I thought, *first the crib pad from the lying-in hospital, and now a washcloth from this place. Collecting cheap mementoes. Stealing. But just a little. They wouldn't miss it and I could use it. Never can tell when you'll run low on things. . . .*

I was back in bed now, tossing, turning, restless.

A nurse came over. 'Mrs. Kruger. Your doctor is here to see you.'

I put on my slippers and walked to the door. He was standing in the hallway.

'How are you, Judith?'

I found myself staring at him because I couldn't remember his face. I had seen him only once before, on the day I was admitted.

'Let's go over here.' He motioned me to a chair. 'How are you feeling?'

'The same. All right. I mean nervous. Very nervous.' I wanted to talk to him, to talk and talk, but I couldn't gather my thoughts.

'The tests were negative.'

'What tests?' I had no recollection of any tests.

'The metabolism studies. And others. There doesn't seem to be anything wrong with your glands.'

I thought, *I knew it all the time. Of course there's nothing wrong with my body. Body. Want to move out of my body. Don't want a body any more.*

'. . . think you can go home now and we'll see what happens . . . the baby. How do you feel about the baby?'

I realized he was waiting for an answer, and I tried to respond. But something was growing inside me—something thick and heavy. And it sat on my chest and I couldn't talk.

He stood up. His body loomed so big. He was a tall man and was well built.

'I have to go now. I'm signing you out. Jay will keep me posted. Your mother is with you?'

'Yes.'

'Good. Try to relax about the baby, will you?'

'Yes.'

I watched him enter the lift. I didn't see him again until September. . . .

Jay came for me the next day, July 12th. I had been in the hospital for just one week. I packed my suitcase with shaking fingers, pushing the washcloth to the bottom where Jay wouldn't notice it.

I sat on a long wooden bench in the Admissions room while Jay took my hospitalization insurance folder to the desk. In a few minutes he came back smiling.

'O.K., sweetie. All clear. Let's go home now.' He took the suitcase and led me out. 'By the way, all we had to pay was forty-seven cents! Imagine! Your insurance covered everything.'

I thought, *that's good. Very good. I wasn't an expense. I'm cheap. I cost him only forty-seven cents. I'm not a burden.*

The hospital was situated in mid-city. There were tall buildings everywhere. I walked close to him and looked up. So tall they were, so big.

So top-heavy. As though they want to topple and crush me, close me in. Everything is closing in. Steel bands on my chest. I can hardly breathe.

As we rode through traffic I became nauseous.

Jay said, 'Our new apartment is only two blocks from my hospital. It was a lucky break that I got it. And I bought some furniture. I think you'll like it, sweetie.'

'Yes. Sure.' I was going home, to a new place, a place I had never seen. Home to my baby, whose face I could barely remember. That tiny, sweet baby who terrified me.

I walked into the apartment as if in a trance. My mother was there, and so was my father. I kissed them mechanically. Jay was cheerful and encouraging. He showed me through the rooms, and I followed him like a frightened child.

My mind tried to encompass the newness and the strangeness, but my eyes focused on only two things. He had put doilies under two lamps he had bought. And in the bedroom I saw the pictures—two eight-by-ten photographs, in plastic frames, of

Jay and myself. He had found them in one of the cartons and had set them up on a dresser. All of the furniture was either second-hand, bought from a storage company, or borrowed from the hospital.

. Our faces in the photos seemed to leap out at me, smiling, happy, composed. I felt as if I were being stabbed.

'Oh, Jay. Take them down . . . The pictures . . . It was so nice of you to put them out, but we don't need them. Jay, we don't need them! (*Pictures and doilies. He tried to make the place look like home. But doilies get dirty and have to be washed and ironed. And pictures. Of us. Of what we were. What I was. Don't want to see myself. Don't want to be.*) 'Jay,' my voice was rising now, 'you'll take them away? Please, please, take them away!'

He looked at me and took my hand. 'O.K. I will. I'll do it now. I'll——'.

'Oh, Jay, Jay!' I crumpled on the bed. 'I'm sick. So sick. I'm afraid. What's wrong with me? What's *wrong*?'

He squeezed my hand. 'I don't know, sweetie. But it'll be all right.'

He didn't know and I didn't know and my parents stood by in helplessness and confusion. Mother took complete care of Gary, but she tried so hard to draw me out and into activity around the house.

'Judith, come. Let's make the formula. See? It's easy. It's just a two-to-one ratio of powder to water. Let's make it together. Get the measuring cup. Now the spoon. I've got the formula. There. You're doing fine. Now see, we add the water. I've boiled it . . .'

Later she would say, 'Help me bathe Gary. Here's the water and soap and towel. He's ready. Oh, is he a doll! You know something funny? We were so busy moving from the other place we nearly forgot him! This darling, and we almost forgot him. He slept for three hours. How's the water? Too cool?'

And I tried. How I tried. I roused myself from the stupor of fear to attempt small chores. I would write outlines of when to feed him, how many vitamin drops for his formula, when to put out rubbish for collection, and on which days the nappy man came. I was trying to hold on to reality with scribblings and jottings and small details. A thousand whens and wheres and whys. I wanted to know everything, to get things under control. But I floundered and dissolved in tears.

'Mom, it's no use,' I cried, 'no use, no use! Look. My hands. They're shaking. I can't stop the shaking.'

And inside, a great fear. And no sleep. I was consuming phenobarbitone and Seconal as if they were aspirin. One night, as I went to shake out three pills, I poured them all into my hand and counted them. Twenty-two pink and whites.

Little pills. Pills for sleep. No good like this, in twos and threes. Suppose I took enough to stop everything. To get a good, long sleep. Oh, God, if I could only sleep!

I set the box back on the shelf and slammed the door of the medicine cabinet. Then I looked at myself in the mirror. I saw a strange face. It was my face, yet it was not. There was nothing behind it that was familiar and right. I stared and asked myself, what's happening to me? What's wrong?

I'm moving back. I'm slipping. A fear so big is pushing me, pressing me, sitting on me. Can't think straight. But I'm not crazy, am I? Am I? Just sick. Very very wrong-sick. Scared-sick. Have to stop it. The pills. Take sleeping pills . . . Easy. No pain. Don't have to hurt my body. Don't want to but have to. Will I have to? When? When I can't breathe or speak any more. When everything closes in.

'Jay. Touch me. Please. Touch me.'

He had just come home. It was the night of July 19th. It was a week since I returned from the hospital.

'What is it, sweetie? My darling? What do you want me to do?' He put his arm round my shoulders.

'Touch me. Hold me. Kiss me. Please.'

'Like this?' He pressed his lips on mine.

'Like before. The way we did before. Caress me. My face. My arms. My body. Please.'

'Why, sweetie?' He was trying to catch my eye, but I wouldn't look at him.

'Because I have no feeling. I'm getting dead inside. Cold and dried up and dead. Touch me again, Jay. Again.'

His hands caressed my body.

'I'm trying. I'm really trying.'

'What are you trying?'

'To feel. To have feeling. But it's no good. I can't feel sex or love or anything. Just dead.'

'You're nervous. You're very upset. You can't expect to feel the same as——'

. I broke from him and ran to the dresser. I pulled out a sheet of paper from the top drawer and handed it to him.

'See this? Read it! I wrote it down. Today. Everything's there.'

I had scrawled the following phrases: 'Cold and dried up inside . . . afraid of winter and rain . . . want to sit in a corner and not talk, not say anything . . . face like a mask, getting tighter and tighter . . . no expression . . . no feeling . . . everything slowing up and running down . . . don't want to touch anything or do anything . . . want to move out of my body and disappear . . . no inner strength . . . afraid of everything . . . of my husband . . . my family . . . my baby . . . want baby but scared of him . . . want to scream when I think of him . . . don't want to live . . . moving farther from reality . . . still talk but less and less willing . . . cold . . . so cold . . . and very very tight . . .'

He put the paper down.

'This is how you feel?'

'Yes. And it's getting worse. Every minute. I want to die.'

My mother walked into the room and heard me speak.

'What are you saying? What are you saying?'

'I want to kill myself. That's all. Simple, isn't it? *Isn't it?*'

My voice rose.

Jay shook his head at her. 'Leave her alone, Frieda. She doesn't mean it.'

'I do. I do mean it.'

Mother's face was drawn and she spoke through tight lips. 'You'll be sorry. So sorry.'

They're warning . . . and threatening . . . And trying to keep me in line. Tell me it's nothing . . . take it easy . . . Are they sick? Are they living in terror? Yesohyes, they mean well when they reassure, but it's no good and it's too late. They can't help and I can't fight any more. Know what I have to do now to stop this closing in.

'Judith?' Mother was speaking softly, pleadingly. 'Come here, please. Help me with the nappies. Go outside in the yard and hang these up for me. Jay put a line up yesterday. Here. Take them.'

I stepped into the back-yard. It was overgrown with weeds and wild grasses. I stumbled on the uneven ground and a clean nappy fell out of my hands. I picked it up and dropped it again. My fingers wouldn't co-ordinate. While I struggled with a few clothes-pins a neighbour came out of her house. I quickly turned my face away. I didn't want anyone to see me. Then another nappy fell. The afternoon sun burned hot on my back. It wanted to blast me, to suffocate me. I crumpled the nappies into a ball and ran back into the house.

'I told you I can't do it!' I screamed to my mother. 'I can't do anything! Everything is falling apart! I can't even hang up three nappies!'

'Don't worry about it. It's all right. It's all right', she said. 'Do something else. Take a cup of coffee. You haven't eaten all day. Or a cold soft drink. It's hot. Take a peach, maybe.'

I looked at her. She was trying so hard, grasping at one thing after another, to keep me occupied. And I felt sorry for her.

'No. I don't want anything to eat. Where's Jay?'

'Back at the hospital. He got an emergency call.'

'I'm going to take a bath.'

'Good. That's fine. You'll cool off and then you'll feel better', she said.

Sitting in the tub, I watched the trembling of my hands and was afraid to use the razor to shave my legs. I stared at the razor and wondered what it would be like to cut my wrists. Does the first slash hurt? And what do you do until the loss of blood makes you faint? Do you stand over the basin and watch the blood drip and try to keep it off the floor where it would make a mess? Or do you lie down and wait? What do you do?

Don't even know the right way to die.

I stepped out of the tub and got into my housecoat. In a moment I was once more dripping with perspiration and my head was filled with the throbbing of my pulse. The fluorescent light in the bathroom glared white, illuminating every object. I looked at my comb and brush, my towels, my talcum powder, my toilet articles, afraid to touch them. They were part of me and I didn't want them.

I wanted to get out. Escape. I had to get away from pain and fear. I didn't want to move or touch. Do nothing. Be nothing. Just be dead. Through the closed door I heard my baby cry, and my stomach knotted in terror. I moved to the medicine cabinet and opened the door.

The sleeping pills. Last time you counted there were twenty-two pills. Take the box. Slide open the cover. There they are. Pink and white. It'll be easy. No blood like with the razor. Just sleep. And that's what you want. Take them. What are you waiting for? I'm waiting because I want to tell them what I'm going to do so they'll know how terrible I feel, how sick I am, and they'll try to stop me but I won't let them. Will I?

I heard the front door slam. Jay was coming down the hall. I flung open the bathroom door and yelled: 'Jay! Jay! I'm taking the pills!'

I grabbed up a handful and swallowed them in twos and threes, gulping water from the tap. He rushed in and grappled with me. I fought to tear away.

'*No* you don't', he said. 'No! No!' His hands closed over my wrists and forced them down. 'Let go, *let go*!'

The pills spilled over the floor.

'See? See?' I was screaming now. 'I want to die!'

Mother ran in and Jay said, 'She took the sleeping pills, Frieda.' His voice cracked.

Her face turned ashen.

'Oh, my God! Judith! I told you. You'll be sorry. You——'

I slumped to the floor, beating my hands against my face. I wanted to speak, to tell them that I had to do it, but my tongue was too big for my mouth. Jay lifted me up. I felt the sweat on his hands. He led me to the bed. But I wouldn't lie there. I got up and staggered through the apartment, past the baby's bassinet. As though from a far distance I heard him crying.

I fell face down on the couch in the living-room.

For the first time in six weeks I slept. But it was only for a few hours. Then I felt someone shaking me. Jay's face was next to mine. And I saw the figures of my parents. But there was someone else squatting in front of me—a small, dark man with a little black moustache.

He spoke. 'Judith, how are you?'

I blinked through drug-laden eyes. 'All right.' I tried to get up, but it was too much of an effort. Sleep. I wanted more sleep. 'Mmn-m-n . . .' I mumbled, and lay back on the couch again, turning my back to everyone.

Jay caught my arm and brought me to a sitting position.

'Judy, sweetie? Listen to me. This is Doctor Edelson . . .'

'Hello', I said, and thought, *why doesn't he get up? Looks so silly squatting there . . . They all look silly. Their heads are big and fuzzy . . . Everything's silly.*

I blinked my eyes.

'. . . all right . . . to the hospital . . . treatment . . . the baby . . . need help . . .' That doctor was talking to me, his voice coming from far away. I barely heard him. I was wrapped in a cottony blanket of sedation. But I tried to concentrate on his words.

'Hospital? What hospital?'

'The State Hospital. You'll get good treatment there. You need some help, Judith. They'll make you well again.'

That was Jay's voice. And there was something white and crackly in his hands. I didn't know it at the time, but while I was sleeping he had gone to see Doctor Downey, who had admitted me to the Philadelphia hospital, and obtained commitment papers from him. The other doctor with me now was a local general practitioner. Commitment to a State hospital requires the signature of two physicians.

The little man got to his feet and seemed to disappear into the background. It was dark in the living-room. I had no idea what time it was.

'When do I go?' No more terror now. Just a numbing dullness.

'Tonight', Jay said. 'It'll be better, sweetie.'

'O.K. Pack. Have to pack, don't I?'

'Yes. Can you stand up?' His arm was strong across my back.

'Think so. Just tired.'

'Sure. I know.'

My parents stepped out from the shadows of the room and my father said, 'I'll go with you, darling.'

'All right, Dad.' And I walked slowly through the hall to the bedroom. My mother followed.

'Mom, how may dresses should I take, huh? Underwear. Shoes? Mom, would you get my blue valise?'

Just unpacked that suitcase from one hospital. Now I'm going to another one. Like one holiday after another. Never a dull moment. Dull . . . feel so dull and dopey and heavy and slow . . . what happened . . . what did I do . . . what . . . oh, yeah . . . took the pills . . . Jay stopped me . . . wanted him to stop me, didn't I? But why? Can't remember now . . . slips . . . should I take this pretty one? Wonder what they wear there? Maybe I'll need very little. Yes. That would be good . . . to wear nothing.

As I opened one drawer after another I saw that my hands were beginning to tremble again. The effect of the sedatives was wearing off.

The baby was sleeping when I tiptoed through his room. I wanted to look at him, but I couldn't. And I had no words for my mother as she stood at the door, looking small and so very worried, and twisting a nappy round and round in her hands.

'I . . . I'm sorry, Mom . . . I . . . I'll see you . . .'

'Yes, sure, darling. Soon.'

Jay drove the car into Philadelphia where we took a midnight bus. It was old and it rattled along the empty roads. I reached for Jay's hand and held it tightly. I wanted to talk to him, to explain away what I had done. But I couldn't frame the words. We stopped once at a diner for a five-minute rest. I sat upright and rummaged through my pocketbook for a pencil and a blank card. I had suddenly remembered a fragment of conversation between Jay and the little doctor when they were standing next to the couch in the apartment. They had used the words 'shock treatments'. I knew little about shock, but I remembered reading some place that it makes you forget things and names and places. So I carefully wrote down my name, my age, my new address, our New York address, the names of members of my family, our telephone number, the baby's name, when and where he was born, plus my Social Security number.

The bus rumbled back on to the highway. My father had the seat behind us, and I remember him touching my shoulder once or twice. Then Jay nudged me.

'Judy? We're here . . . I've got your suitcase. Can you get up?'

'Yes.'

I stumbled after him out of the bus. The night was cool and damp and I shivered. My father hailed a taxi. As we stepped into it fear swept through me like a fire. Now I was fully awake, and tense again, and afraid.

Go back. Hold back. Tell them you won't go. Don't want to go. Fight them. Run away.

But it was too late for entreaties. I had made the decision for them when I swallowed the pills.

It was only a short ride from the bus stop to the hospital. Darkness closed in as the street lights became less frequent. Then I saw trees, tall and black. Then a gate outlined by a yellow light burning above it.

'All right, sweetie. We're here.'

My father took my hand and squeezed it and I felt his fear, too—his reluctance to accept what I had done and where I was going. He and Jay helped me out. I was very cold now. Crickets were chirping in the grass as we walked up a path to a grey stone building. A door opened and two nurses, their uniforms chalky-white, stepped out to meet us.

I felt Jay press my hand and then the brush of his lips on my cheek. Then my father was next to me and there was something wet in his eyes. The nurses were closer now. Jay handed them my suitcase. Then one of them grasped my arm under the elbow. Now there was a nurse on each side of me. I turned my head, but Jay and my father were gone. It was black behind me, and the crickets were screaming.

Why did I let them . . . don't want to be here . . . shouldn't have let them . . . want to go home now . . . have to go home . . . what did I do did I do did I DO?

Terror washed over me in waves. I couldn't raise my head to look at the nurses. I walked between them, watching the toes of their shoes. They led me to a lift. A clanging and a whirring and a door squealing shut and then opening. And then there were noises and voices, and hands upon me, stripping off my clothes, turning me, wrapping me in a short nightgown open at the back. Then they put me in a bed that was high and white.

Now I had to look because of the light. So much light, glaring from the ceiling. And so much noise. Like a babble and a roar and a cry and a wail.

I was in the Women's General Admissions ward of the State Hospital. Every newly-admitted patient was sent here. It was a huge room, and most of the beds were occupied. But some of the women were sitting on chairs at the foot of the beds, or walking barefoot up and down the aisles.

I hunched in the corner of my bed and stared.

God oh God, I'm in a crazy house. What'll they do to me? What'll they do? I'm the new one . . . the newest . . . and they're watching me . . . which one'll hit me and hurt me first? I'm scared. Oh, God, I'm scared . . . There . . . that one there with the hair hanging down and the funny eyes . . . why doesn't she get into bed and stop that pacing? . . . and there's another . . . squatting like an Indian and talking to herself. They're all talking and I can't hear them . . . can't understand them . . . what are they saying . . . are they talking about me? Why don't the nurses come . . . something could happen . . . so many of them . . . they could gang up and rush to my bed and I can't move I'm so scared . . . There! See? I knew it! One's coming now . . . right to me . . . maybe she's got a knife . . . where's the nurse . . . oh, please, God, don't let her hurt me.

'Hello.'

A thin, fair woman with a pockmarked face came over to my bed.

'You just came in, didn't you?' She spoke pleasantly.

'Y-yes.'

'I've been here two days now.'

'Y-you don't look sick', I said. 'I mean——'

'I am. It's my stomach. I can't eat anything. I'm here for observation. But I don't think they'll find anything. The other doctors didn't. I've been to three hospitals, and none of them know what's wrong with me. Well, I'll see you. I have to get some sleep.'

'You sleep here? With all the lights on?'

'You'll get used to it; you'll see.' She walked away towards the other end of the room.

I turned my face to the wall and closed my eyes, then opened them quickly. Someone was standing next to my bed making soft clucking sounds. It was a buxom Negro woman. Her face was moon-shaped under a stocking cap knotted round her head. Her full bosom strained against her thin cotton dress as she leaned over and touched my arm.

'Tch, tch, there—how ye be?' she said, in a low, crooning voice. 'Gonna git ye some juice, honey', and then she was gone. She returned in a few minutes carrying a plastic cup filled with some fruit juice. She cocked her head to one side as she watched me drink. Then she patted my back for a few moments. Her fingers felt rough and callused, but the steady rhythm was comforting.

'Now git yerself some rest, honey', she murmured. Then she tucked in the sheets and waddled away.

Soon a nurse came by and shut off the overhead lights. I lay rigid in the bed listening to the snuffles and the cries, the giggling and the sudden bursts of laughter.

Now they'll get me! Now they're coming! They'll walk like cats in their bare feet. They'll sneak up and choke me or slash me. Oh, Jay, Jay, you made a mistake. A terrible mistake. Why did you send me here? You thought you did right, but it's wrong. I'm worse. Worse than before. Now I'm scared for real. There are crazy people here. And I'm not crazy, I'm sick! I'll never get well here, Jay.

'Oh, my God!' I cried out. Someone had touched my arm. It was a nurse.

'Put your slippers on, Judith.' She pointed to the floor at a pair of muslin slippers. 'Doctor Manning wants to see you.'

She led me off the ward and down a hall to a small office. A tall, thin man was sitting at a desk, one leg crossed high on the other.

The doctor. Is this my doctor? His face . . . so thin and dark. I'm afraid of him.

The nurse sat me down at the side of the desk. I shivered in the flimsy nightgown. He stared at me and I dropped my eyes. When he spoke his voice was cool and sharp.

'Well, Judith. Are you going to try it again?'

'I—I—don't under . . .' Then I realized he referred to my suicide attempt.

'Oh, no. No, Doctor Manning. I promise. I'm just so sick and I don't know what's wrong with me. I tried to show them how terrible I feel. I just tried. . . . Oh, please, Doctor, I'm so nervous here. So afraid. This place is making me worse. The patients . . . I'm so frightened of them . . . I've never been in a mental hospital before. Take me out of here. Please!'

'Why does it bother you?'

'Why? Because I . . . I . . . I'm not just ordinary. I'm not crazy. I'm . . . I'm educated. I went to college. I don't know how this could happen to me.'

He didn't answer. My words echoed back in my ears and I thought, *Stupid, stupid. Why did you tell him that? What the hell does Phi Beta Kappa mean here? Now he'll think you're really crazy!*

I tried to look at him, to read an answer in his eyes, but I was too ashamed. I sat with my hands in my lap while he asked me a few more questions about my husband and baby. I wanted to answer rationally and calmly, but with each reply I repeated how the ward added to my fears and would he please transfer me. He made no response.

The nurse brought me back to my bed. I twisted from side to side in uncontrollable restlessness.

'All right, Judith. Get up. You're going to Ward A.'

The same nurse was back. I heard her words and jumped out of the bed and shuffled after her to the lift.

Transferred. Thank God. He's good, that Manning. He understood me. He's taking me out of here.

Ward A occupied the entire first floor of the building I had entered. A door led from the hall into a large room called the Day Room. It had tables, chairs, a television set mounted on the wall, and windows that faced the hospital grounds. The patients spent most of the day there, reading, writing, and playing cards and games.

They had no room for me in any of the main wards. The nurse took me into a spare room next to the nursing office. It had a bed, a dressing-table with a mirror, and a storage cabinet. There was something else in the room, on the floor. The nurse had taken my glasses away and in the half-light of the dawn I couldn't see too well. It was a large, flat bundle that looked like a pile of laundry.

I lay in the high bed, hearing the voices from the nursing office, and the first shrill calls of the birds outside. Suddenly, the room was swarming with patients, all of them wearing the short open-backed nightgowns. I jumped out of bed and backed into a corner of the small room.

A woman in a blue uniform came in and opened the big flat bag and all the women huddled round it, pulling and grabbing, and coming up with rolled bundles of clothing. They pulled out lettered tongue depressors, laid them on the dressing-table, and shook out their clothing. Then they stripped off their nightgowns and dressed. I stared at their nakedness.

Then someone else dressed in a blue uniform pushed into the room and called my name.

'Kruger? You here?'

'Yes. Here I am.' I could barely see her behind the crowd of women. She manœuvred her way through them and dumped a bundle on the dressing-table.

'Here's your clothes. Roll call in ten minutes.'

Then she pushed her way out, calling over her shoulder, 'Hurry up, girls. Hurry up!'

The patients drifted out. I was fumbling with the buttons at the back of my dress when a grey-haired nurse bustled in with a pile of sheets in her arms.

'Hello, Judith. How are you, honey?' She stripped my bed and made it up with fresh linen, pulling the sheets smooth and taut. She had a small, pink face. 'I'm Mrs. Hendricks. I'm on night duty. I'm going off in a few minutes. I know you just came in and I wanted to say hello. I hope you're feeling all right.'

I wanted to please her because she looked like everybody's grandmother and spoke so kindly. But I couldn't.

'I'm sick, Mrs. Hendricks. Very sick. And I'm afraid here.'

'Now, now.' She patted my hand. 'Don't say that. There's nothing to be afraid of, and you're going to get well. Then you'll go home to your husband and your baby.' She gathered up the soiled linen and left.

I wondered how she knew about me. They all seemed to know my name, that I was married, and had a baby. I went to the doorway, but she had disappeared. I stood blinking and squinting at the activity in the hall. Nurses were going back and forth through a door at the end of the hall. They were carrying

3

trays on which I saw hypodermic syringes and rubber tubes and large pitchers. A few patients trailed in and out of the hall, some carrying towels and toothbrushes. They went into the bathroom opposite my room, then pattered back to the room behind the door.

I didn't know it at this time, but insulin shock treatment was already under way for the patients in that ward. Each day, five times a week, they were wakened at five-thirty a.m. Insulin shock requires a long procedure, and a staff of specially trained nurses prepare the patients for the injection of the drug, supervise the successive stages of the induced coma, and administer sugar to counteract the insulin and bring them out of coma.

I remained standing in the corridor until a nurse approached me and gave me my glasses.

'Here,' she said, 'we kept them in the office last night because you came in so late. Tonight they'll go in the regular place.'

What is the regular place? And what do I do now? And where do I go? And what and when and why?

My chest was bursting with unspoken questions. I was in a strange and frightening place. I wanted to get out, but I was in and no one was telling me anything. Why didn't they give me a little booklet, neatly bound, and headed, 'Guide to Your State Hospital'? Something to read, to learn, to cling to.

Orientation came slowly and painfully. I grasped hungrily at each facet of routine.

I put on my glasses. Doors and hallways sprang into sharp focus. And I heard better, too.

'Roll call. Into the Day Room, everyone.'

'Kruger! You! Come on!' An attendant took my arm and led me to the big room with all the tables and chairs. Patients were pouring in from both entrances. In the middle of the room stood a blue-uniformed woman with a notebook resting on her arm. The clock in the corridor said six-forty-five a.m. I sat down in a chair next to a thin girl with glasses, as the attendant started the roll call. The girl leaned towards me.

'Did you just come in?' Her voice was thin and trembly.

'Yes. Last night.'

'My name is Beverly Vaughn. I don't like it here. I'm afraid here. Are you afraid?'

'Yes. I was never in a place like this before.' As I spoke to her, her eyes filled with tears.

'I don't know what's going to happen to me. Nobody cares. I pray a lot. I wish I had my Bible. What's your name?'

'Judith Kruger.'

'Will you be my friend, Judith?'

I was embarrassed by her blunt and open pleading and that beaten look in her eyes. 'Yes, I'll be your friend.'

'Kruger? Kruger?' The blue lady was calling my name.

'Here!' My voice sounded strange and too loud.

Patients were still drifting in. More names, more answering voices, and then, 'All right, everyone. Cafeteria! Cafeteria!'

Two more nurses appeared and herded us out of the Day Room, through another large ward with many beds, and along a short hall with a locked door at the end. Beverly was still at my side.

'We have to wait until it's time for our ward. We go to cafeteria at seven.'

I lifted my arm to look at my watch. It wasn't there. I started in fear. My rings were gone too. Wedding ring and school ring. Then I remembered giving them to Jay before we said good-bye. Was it only five hours ago?

Cautiously I let my eyes shift from one face to another as we stood in a weaving line. And once, quickly, I turned right round to see the end of the line. There were about fifty of us.

All sick? I thought. *Sick like me? How long have they been here, and why? Did they try to kill themselves the way I did? Are they as scared as I am? Do they sleep at night? Do they worry?*

'Let's go, girls!' The attendant rattled a bunch of keys hanging from her belt and unlocked the door. I was pushed from behind into a square hall. Suddenly a terrific stench assailed me.

'Beverly . . . that smell! God, what is it?' She pulled me along, pointing to an open archway in the middle of the hall. From an opposite door elderly women were shuffling slowly. They were bringing the foulness with them, the odours of urine, of excrement, of incontinence and despair. The smell of impending death.

I hurried on. We moved up a sloping ramp. To the right, down a stairway, rushed a horde of women, their feet clattering on the iron steps. The sound echoed back twenty years to public school and Auditorium day. Dressed in starched middies, red ties, and navy skirts, we poured out of our classrooms and clambered down the stairways, the heels of our polished shoes thundering on the corrugated treads. Then the line by the Auditorium doors. And the march down the aisle as the piano pounded 'Come Let Us Walk In-To the Spring While the Dum-De-Dumm Dum Dum-de Sing'. The women rushing past wore blue too. Faded, torn blue dresses. Were they dresses or sacks? No collars or sleeves or belts. I thought, is that what they give them to wear? How awful! But I looked again and saw wild staring eyes and streaming hair, lips contorted and mumbling. I flattened myself against the wall.

The large cafeteria was divided into two sections by a railing. Male patients ate on one side, women on the other. On our side there were at least two nurses on duty, stationed at the entrance and at the check-out spot where we left our trays and utensils. The food was plain but hot; portions were small but we were allowed 'seconds' if we took our tray back to the steam table.

I moved away from the serving area and scanned the tables, which were filling up fast. I tried to look for Beverly or the other women from my ward, but all the faces looked unfamiliar. I was afraid to sit down with strangers. Maybe they'd hit me, or curse me, or throw food at me. Actually, they did none of these things. Eating hours were uneventful and incidents were rare. But sometimes an accident occurred, and it did that morning. As I moved between the tables a young girl passed by me. Suddenly she fell to the floor with a gurgling cry, and her tray clattered down. I stared, frozen, at the blood welling from a cut on her head. Her tongue hung from her mouth, her eyes rolled upward, and her body writhed in slow convulsions. A nurse pushed me aside, signalled to the check-out nurse, and together they turned her over on her side. I collapsed into the nearest empty chair, unable to look back at the figure on the floor.

The woman opposite lifted her fork and pointed behind me. 'Fit. That one ain't so bad. She gets them worse, sometimes. You should see.' She stabbed her bread with the fork, swished it round in the gravy on her plate, and stuffed it in her mouth.

I should see. Yes, I should see. I see and I don't want to. See. Or be or feel. Or know these people and this place. I want to get out of here. Please, God, I want to get out.

I picked up my tray with the food untouched and walked to the check-out section. A male attendant was standing by the large wooden box where the patients deposited their trays and utensils.

I stared at the knife on my tray. Suppose I hid it? But where? My pocket wasn't deep and I had no stockings on. Anyway, it didn't look sharp enough to cut. Or hurt. Or rip open flesh. My flesh.

I dropped the knife into the box and walked on, out of the cafeteria, up the ramp and through the door to my ward. An attendant was standing there with the Roll Book. 'Kruger. Check.' Her wrist-watch said seven-thirty. Another day had begun for the patients of Ward A.

I walked round aimlessly. Many of the women were sloshing mops across the tile floors. Others were scrubbing the bathroom sinks, or making beds. And some were washing down the walls of the Day Room.

Who the hell wants to scrub and work like that? They won't get me to do that kind of stuff.

'That's what they do here every morning.'

I turned. Beverly was standing beside me. Good God, she's so creepy-quiet, I said to myself. Like a wraith.

'We also take out the garbage.'

'Garbage too?'

'Yes. She does it.' She pointed to a husky blonde patient standing by a side door and hefting a pail to her shoulder. It was a large pail, filled with papers and rubbish. She waited by the door until the attendant came to unlock the door and waited while the woman carried the pail down a short flight of steps, emptied it into a metal crate, and then came back to the Day Room.

'She doesn't talk', Beverly said.

'What do you mean?'

'She doesn't say anything. Only when she's angry. Then she curses. I'm afraid of her. Stay away from her.'

'What's her name?'

'Hunter. Josephine Hunter.'

Josephine walked past us to get a mop and a pail nearby. I backed away, remembering Beverly's warning, and stared at her retreating legs. They were large, over-muscled, and covered with heavy blonde hairs. In the next two months I heard Josephine speak only once. We were waiting to go to cafeteria. Someone spoke to her and suddenly she grunted, gritted her teeth, and spewed out a stream of mumbled curses. Then she grabbed the footrail of the nearest bed and banged it down with a crash. We scattered like flies.

'Hunter! You cut that out, now.' An attendant moved in towards her. I flinched, expecting her to be struck, but nothing happened. Josephine made a few more guttural sounds and sat down heavily on the bed, staring dully straight ahead.

I swallowed hard.

It's like living with an animal. A tiger or an ape. She's dangerous. One day she may run amok. Why do they let her stay here with us? She could hurt somebody. Me. I'm afraid.

The sight of all the patients working so busily that first morning made me sick at my stomach. And I had had no breakfast. I went back to the utility room where I had slept the night before. The bed was made up and the room was neat, except for the big bundle of nightclothes sticking out from under the bed.

My nightgown's in there, and I hate it. It has no buttons at the back.

Quickly, I opened the cabinet drawers and rummaged through them. Sheets. Small towels. I stuffed one in the pocket of my dress. And then I grew panicky. Where were all my clothes? Underwear, shoes, dresses, toilet articles. All the things I had packed in my valise.

Why don't they tell me where they are? I've got to find them. I must have my things. Things, things, THINGS!

I threw myself on the bed and clenched my fists until the nails pierced the flesh. Pain. Hurt myself. Good. Do it some more. *More.* I sat up, wringing my hands and pulling at the fingers, trying to wrench them from their sockets. The sound of footsteps made me stop.

A woman came in. She was dressed in a flowered housedress with white ruffles on the neck and pocket. She was soft and plump. She looked like a busy housewife coming in to straighten up a room. I sat and watched her. She went to the mirror over the bureau, and took a lipstick from her pocket and carefully made up her lips. Then she spoke to me in a husky voice.

'You came last night, didn't you?'

'How do you know?'

She shrugged a little. 'We know. When you're here for a while you'll notice new patients, too.'

'Do you know what happened to my clothes?'

She turned back to the mirror. 'I guess they're being stamped in the marking room. Then they send them down here and they put them in the closets.'

'Where are the closets?'

'Two of them are out there.' She pointed through the door to the corridor. 'There's another one in the ward beyond the Day Room.'

'Real closets?' The thought of a private place for my clothes excited me.

'No. Rooms with shelves. Like bins. They keep your clean things there. We get showers twice a week. They take your dirty clothes and give them to your people on visiting days. Your folks take them home and wash them and bring them back the next time. See?'

'Yes. Oh, yes.' Marking room, bins, showers, visiting days. I was so grateful for her explanation that tears came to my eyes. She watched me through the mirror and said, 'Don't be afraid. You'll be all right. You'll get better.'

'But I can't give my clothes to my folks. My mother can't wash them. She's too busy. She has my baby. I just had a baby. It's six weeks old.'

'You can wear state clothes if you want to. Lots of us do.'

'What are "state clothes"?'

'The hospital has plenty of dresses. They give them to women who don't have a family. Or who are poor. This dress is mine.' She patted the ruffled pocket. 'But I have only a few. Most of the time I wear state clothes. You have a little baby. Your first?'

'Yes. That's why I'm here. Something happened to me when he was born. I'm afraid of him. I'm afraid of everything.'

'I have twelve children.'

'Oh, my God! You have?'

She laughed in the same husky way she spoke. 'Twelve nice kids and one terrible husband. I don't live with him any more.'

'Where are your children?'

'Relatives. Welfare agencies. Around. Most of them are grown up. I'm thirty-eight—I got married young.'

'You look young.'

'Thank you. I was very sick when I came here. I had shock.'

'Shock?'

'Insulin shock. I'm finished now. I'm on parole. I can go out on the grounds. I help the nurses and work in the laundry. But I have to stay here until Social Service finds me a job and gets my family fixed up. I can't take the younger ones back. There's no money. My husband left me. He was a bad man. He forced me and made me pregnant all the time.' She sighed. 'But I don't think much about it now. You see I'm better.' She walked to me and put her hand on mine. It was rough and warm. 'You'll get better, too, and you'll go home to your baby. I have to go now and fold some clothes. Do you want to help?'

'No. Not yet. Later, maybe.'

'All right, I'll see you. My name is Anna. What's yours?'

'Judith.'

'Good-bye, Judy.'

I jumped off the bed and watched her walk down the corridor and then turn out of sight. As I stood in the doorway a young Negro attendant approached.

'You Kruger?'

She was small and wiry and looked about nineteen. She wore brown-and-white saddle shoes.

'Yes.'

'Your clothes are here. And you got a cabinet in the other ward. I'll show you where I put your things.' A row of white steel cabinets lined each side of the ward at the far end of the Day Room. 'You're over there. I just inked the tape, so don't smudge it. See you.'

My name was printed in large block letters on a strip of adhesive tape. Another strip was under mine. Evidently I would share this cabinet with some other patient. Inside were my make-up kit, talcum powder, soap, a box of notepaper,

pencils, and my wallet. I opened it. It was empty of money but
contained the little card on which I had written my name,
address, and the name of my baby. My hands shook as I stared
at it. I turned the card face down and shoved it back in the
wallet. Then I took out the little towel I had stolen from the
utility room and stuffed it into the back of my shelf.

Morning clean-up was over. Patients were drifting in and out
of the ward. Some of them lay down on the beds, but nurses and
attendants who were passing through kept prodding them to
get up.

'C'mon, girls. No lying on beds. Get up. Off the beds, everybody!'

In the middle of the ward was a door through which patients
were going in and out. I edged over and looked in. This was the
bathroom and the shower room. It smelled of wet floors,
cigarette smoke, and urine. I had to urinate badly that first
morning and I waited for the crowd to thin out. But as soon as
a few drifted away more came in to occupy the toilets and the
floor. I walked in, saw the open toilets, and flushed with embarrassment. But no one paid the slightest attention to me. The
only private places in A Ward were the isolation rooms with
their tiny barred windows and their padded walls.

I sat on the toilet and thought of a conversation I had had
with Jay shortly after his release from the Navy.

'*You mean, the bathrooms had no doors? Weren't you embarrassed?*'

'*At first I was, but then you get used to it and you don't care. You
can get used to anything.*'

That was how it was with us in A Ward . . . after a while we
just didn't care. Much more important were the rumours
picked up in the bathroom about treatment and doctors and
release dates. Salesgirls huddle and talk of tally sheets and
commissions. Waitresses compare tips. Housewives trade recipes
and compare meat prices. But here they used strange words.
Words like 'shock' and 'solitary' and 'O.T.' and 'secondarys',
'spinals', 'coma', 'Staff', and 'parole'.

A tall, middle-aged woman was talking loudly in the centre
of a group near the window. She used her lighted cigarette as a
teacher would use a blackboard pointer.

'I've been shocked and un-shocked and re-shocked and

de-shocked', she yelled. 'When the hell they going to stop? I got more shock than anyone in this goddam place. I got the world's record for shock.' She dropped the cigarette in the toilet and started to laugh.

'Esther, you're funny', someone said.

'Yeah. Funny like this shit-house is funny. Some mornings I wake up I don't know my own name.'

The women nodded and clucked in sympathy. They looked as if they really were sorry for her. But I soon learned how fragile and fleeting are the friendships in a mental hospital. There were very few who made strong emotional attachments. Normal motivations were lacking. Every scrap of information gleaned from huddled conversation was translated in terms of self. A patient who cared more for a friend's welfare than her own was viewed with suspicion and fear. That was how it was with Theresa Coppola. She attached herself to the most helpless patient on the ward, and all the other patients, including myself, were afraid to criticize her.

Theresa was only seventeen, but her behaviour and mannerisms were those of a woman four times her age. She was short and stocky, with sharp black eyes, and she wore her straight hair in heavy bangs. She had spent one year in a convent school and always folded down the collar of her dress to show the large cross that hung from her neck. Her rimless glasses and the hard, tight expression she wore made me think of a stern headmistress in a girls' school who brooks no laughter or sacrilegious word.

Theresa was admitted to A Ward two days after I was, and her first contacts were not with the patients but with the nurses. She dogged their heels, asking for work. She helped make up the beds, took charge of morning clean-up, straightened the Day Room, and hung around the nursing office waiting for errands. As soon as she felt secure with the staff, she shifted her authority to the patients. If one of us lay down on a bed, Theresa would stand there clucking and shaking her head. She walked through the wards commenting on the dusting and the mopping, and every morning she would check the wards to round up the laggards for roll call. She never lingered in the washroom because she hated smoke and cigarettes and lipstick and

primping and 'gab-gab-gab'. I was afraid to talk when Theresa
was near. She might report me to a nurse or an attendant. A
few of the women said she could read our thoughts.

We were all relieved when Theresa found her special soul to
save. Nancy Kile, at thirteen, had been at State for more than
half her life. A severe attack of measles had produced encepha-
litis, causing permanent brain damage. Her body was beautiful,
with fulling breasts and long firm thighs. Thick hair, chestnut
brown, fell to her waist. Her blue eyes were large and flecked
with grey. But they were mirrors of emptiness. Nancy couldn't
talk except for an occasional whimper or grunt. She couldn't
dress herself or eat with utensils or hold a pencil. Yet she smiled.
All day she smiled with those cherry lips and blue-grey eyes.
She was the pet of the ward and the nurses took pleasure in
keeping her neat and changing her clothes and braiding the
thick plaits of her hair. She slept in her own room—one of the
isolation rooms fixed up with a cot and a rocking chair and
picture books and little stuffed toys.

This was Nancy, and Theresa was irresistibly drawn to her.
She mothered and smothered her with a fierce and hungry
affection, jealous of anyone who offered casual attention. She
would wake her in the morning, dress her, and braid her hair.
She rushed through her breakfast in the cafeteria to come back
to the Day Room, where she supervised Nancy's breakfast.
She hovered over the child like a lioness, ready to claw at
outsiders.

About a month later Theresa was transferred to another
ward. None of us liked her and we were all glad she was gone,
but we wondered about Nancy. Was there a sense of sadness
and loss? Did she really hug her Teddy bear tighter, or was it
just our imagination?

By late afternoon of that first day, panic had risen like a gorge
in my throat. I was sitting at the end table in the Day Room.
A young woman with horn-rimmed glasses and curly brown
hair was bent over a jigsaw puzzle, selecting and inserting the
little cardboard pieces in solemn concentration.

I swallowed and cleared my throat. 'Can I try with you?'

She looked up and stared blankly, neither accepting nor
rejecting me.

'If you want.' And she lowered her head. I watched her manipulate the pieces and then reached for one near her arm. My hand was shaking so badly I couldn't move it across the table to the half-finished puzzle. A fog of fear clouded my eyes. *. Nothing is the same. Nothing right. Nothing fits. Not even puzzles. Can't do puzzles. Can't do anything. All wrong inside. All wrong, all wrong.*

I dropped the jigsaw piece and clenched my fists. I felt I was drowning in an ocean of fear. I forced myself up and walked through the Day Room, out into the hall, then into an empty ward. I fell on a bed in the corner and turned my face to the wall.

'Judy?'

Beverly was standing there.

'I thought you were sleeping.'

'I can't sleep. I'm sick. I'm so sick. And nobody understands. Nobody cares.'

'God cares. Pray to Him, Judy. Pray to God for help.'

'I can't. I can't do anything.'

'He helped me.' She lay down on the adjoining bed, her head on her folded arm.

'How does God help you when you're sick like us?'

'I don't know how. I just feel better when I pray. Do you know I have a child? A little girl.'

'That's nice.'

'I'm not married. He said he was going to marry me. He was much older. I believed him because I was lonely. I never had boy friends.'

'What happened to the baby?'

'My sister adopted her. She's eight years old now. They live in Texas. I have a brother, too. He's a physicist. He's very smart and wonderful. He lives in North Carolina. He wrote me a letter. Here. Read it.' She thrust a crumpled envelope into my hand. I made a pretence of reading it.

'Nice. Very nice', I mumbled.

She lay back on the bed with the letter folded on her thin flat chest. Thick tears rolled down her cheeks. 'My brother calls me Bev.' Then she sat up, stuffed the letter in her pocket and walked out of the ward.

She didn't say, 'I'll see you later', or 'Good-bye', or even 'I'm going'. There was no formal conversation here. We spoke only when we wanted to and stopped talking when there was nothing more to say. Disorganized minds shun pretence and politeness.

At four o'clock the attendants went through the wards rounding up the patients for supper. The summer sun slanted through the barrel windows of the Day Room.

'It's so early, isn't it? I mean, for supper.' I spoke to the girl next to me as we moved along the back ward to the locked door leading to the cafeteria.

'Yes. You get hungry later on. But they give us our food packages at night.'

'Packages?'

'On visiting days your family can bring you things. You know—fruit, candy, stuff like that. Some of us get lots. Some don't get anything. They don't have families. Know what I mean?'

'Yes.' And I thought of my father sitting behind me in the bus, his hand gripping the handrail. Was it only last night? And my mother clutching a wadded-up nappy as she stood at the door of the apartment. And Jay. I could still feel the strong pressure of his hand on mine as the taxicab drove up to the hospital. Their faces swam in a painful confusion of need and rejection. And starkly white through the blur of images loomed the bassinet and the tiny figure of my baby. . . .

It was eight o'clock. I was standing in the corridor. The night-shift attendants were herding patients out of the Day Room and straightening the chairs. Women were swarming into the utility room where I had slept the night before. A nurse was pulling open the huge bundle of nightclothes and the patients wriggled out of their clothes and wrapped themselves in the short white nightgowns.

Young bodies, with full firm breasts and buttocks. Old bodies, fat and shapeless. Flesh and form shuffling back and forth, in and out of the room. I saw them roll up their clothes in tight little bundles, slip their name sticks in the knot and drop them on the open sheet. From the bathrooms on each side of the hall I heard the sound of running water. Some of the women were washing out their socks and underwear, draping them on the shower rods.

'You Judith Kruger?' A short and very fat nurse came over to me.

'Yes?'

'Don't look so scared.' Her full face crinkled in a smile.

'I don't have a nightgown. Where am I going to sleep? Last night I was there.' I pointed to the utility room.

'Don't worry about it. C'mere.' Her voice was strong and husky. She led me to a small room next to the nursing office. A long table and many chairs seemed to fill the room. She motioned for me to sit down, and plumped herself into a swivel chair. Then she slid three packets of cigarettes across the polished table. 'Go ahead. Take them. I had to lock up the rest of the carton you had in your suitcase. You're not supposed to have cigarettes, you know.'

'I know.'

'You can smoke now. Go ahead. Smoke.' She lit one of her own cigarettes.

I fumbled with the cellophane tape. 'Thank you, Miss . . .?'

'Mrs. Matthews. I'm on the night shift. Eight to four. What's the matter with you, Judith?' The tiny starched cap bobbled on her fluffy red hair.

'I don't know. I'm just sick and nervous. Terribly nervous. I'm afraid of everything. I just had a baby.'

'They told me you took sleeping pills. Why?'

'I want to die.'

'That was a wrong thing to do. You don't want to die. I have a baby too. He's a year. I don't want to leave him. You listen to me. You keep hold on yourself. You're going to be O.K., you hear?'

She stubbed out her cigarette and stood up, hiking down her girdle. 'I got to get on duty. Now get a nightgown from the attendant and go to bed. You can sleep in the same place as last night. And stop worrying about every little thing.'

Words of rebuttal rushed to my lips but never came out. How could she understand, standing there so squat and easy, so brusquely confident? She touched my shoulder as we stepped

out of the room. 'You're going to be all right. Do you believe
me?'

'Oh, yes. Yes', I lied. 'And thank you, Mrs. Matthews.'

The next morning I tried suicide again.

The night had been long. I had tossed and thrashed on my
bed listening to the muffled voices of the nurses in the nearby
office. I heard feet shuffling along the corridor and toilets
flushing and the sobs of patients from the ward. Suddenly I sat
up in bed and clutched the sheet as a piercing scream tore
through the night. First one, then another and yet another.

Will it never stop? Make it stop, somebody, make it stop!

I remembered the wild-eyed women panting up the cafeteria
ramp. Was it one of them? There are so many here.

*There it goes again. Stop it. Give her a shot or a pill. Sleeping pills.
I want them. Why don't they give you something to let you sleep?* . . .

It was Sunday. Visiting hours were from nine to eleven in the
morning. Two hours to sit with relatives. To ask and answer
questions with hungry eyes. To give thank-yous for the food and
letters. Two hours to shift and squirm in the seats, fiddling with
string from opened packages. To whisper private secrets
momentarily free of mail censorship. Time to search tense and
drawn faces and forced little smiles. Hands held tight across the
table, as if to bridge the gulf between. Voices that crack and
choke with unshed tears. Eyes that dart nervously to watches.
And then the sharp pain of good-bye.

I had no visitors that first Sunday, but I didn't expect any. I
knew Jay was on duty at the hospital and I had been here less
than twenty-four hours. I was actually relieved with the lack
of company because now I wouldn't have to lie and cry to
people, even my own. All they could give was sympathy, and it
wasn't enough.

At ten minutes to eleven the nurses walked through the Day
Room, tapping patients on the shoulder and smiling at the
visitors. 'Visiting hours are over . . . I'm sorry . . . time to go.'
Then they stood to one side, hearing last frenzied bursts of
conversation, watching lips brush cheeks in clumsy kisses, hand
clasp hand for long seconds. 'Next week . . . Bye . . . don't
forget . . . next week.'

It was over. The lift leading to the Day Room clanged shut on the last visitor. Attendants rearranged chairs, swept up bits of newspaper and string and crumbs of food. Everything was as before.

'Who wants to go outside, girls? It's nice out there today.'

I had never seen the woman who spoke to us. She was a light-skinned Negro in a white uniform with a small blue emblem on her breast pocket. Later I found out that the emblem signified a psychiatric technician who had completed a specialized course of training in hospital work. Her status was between that of attendant and nurse.

She was very pretty. Her skin was creamy-brown and her hair curled softly round her ears. As she walked past me I smelled soap and a light cologne. She stood at the door of the Day Room. 'Who's ready to go outside?' She spoke in a high, clear voice. 'There's a nice sun out there, girls.'

I hated the sun. I hung back as the women lined up in front of her. But it was something to do. I moved into the line.

'Twenty-three, twenty-four, twenty-five', she sang out. She opened the door and a cool breeze swept into the room. As I came up to her she looked at me and smiled. 'Hello, Judy. How are you? I'm Miss Willems.'

We walked down the stone steps. I was the last one out. As I came off the steps and on to the grass I saw a large cardboard rubbish box stuffed with package wrappings and newspapers. A long red ribbon dangled from the top of the heap. My eye followed it down to the ground. There was something there glinting in the sun. Glass. Pieces of glass.

'Judy?' Miss Willems was calling me. I looked up and saw the rest of the group about twenty-five feet away hurrying towards benches under a big tree. I caught up with them. Perspiration was bathing my underarms and thighs. I smiled weakly at her and found an empty spot and sat down. Matches flickered feebly in the sun as the patients lit cigarettes. I was trembling too much to smoke. I clung to the iron railing of the bench and stared past the faces of the women sitting round me.

Ring around the rosy, pocket full of posy, all fall down. Run to the glass, pick up the glass, cut with the glass and all fall down. Sick, sick, got to die.

I moved my head slowly. Miss Willems at the next bench fingering her keys. Two girls lying on the grass. Four girls playing cards by a table under the tree. Pine trees, thick and green, poking into the yellow-blue sky. A ribbon road winding down a rise of ground. A Ward building in back. Another one over to the right. And one more behind that.

The door to our building opened and a nurse stood at the top of the steps. She cupped her hands over her mouth and called out something. It sounded like 'Chapel'.

Miss Willems stood up. 'Who wants to go to services? It's Sunday, girls.'

About ten women got up and started across the grass to the steps. Then two more, and then another one.

Now. Now. Go with them. My muscles tensed, but I was frozen to the seat. *They'll stop me. Sunday services are for Gentiles. They must know I'm Jewish. Yet . . . if I run . . .*

'Wait! Me. I'm going to chapel.' I rushed from the seat and ran towards the building, my feet moving without conscious will. There, on the ground, just where I had seen it before. I grabbed a thick chunk of glass. A hand—was it mine?—moved to my throat. Glass against skin. A ripping and a slashing and a screaming. And then the sun was black. . . .

I regained consciousness as they were carrying me through the Day Room. Not dead, I thought, and no pain. For the second time, I had failed in an act of suicide.

I'm sick. And I want to get out. Through a Death-Not-Final. A little here. A little there. A gesture of despair. How else can I prove it to them?

I shut my eyes to the faces lining the Day Room. Shame flushed my cheeks. I wanted to call out, 'Ladies, put me down. I'm all right. I'm sorry for the fuss. I just wanted to try something. Forget it, will you?'

'Oh, for heaven's sake, another one!' I recognized the voice of the head nurse, Mrs. O'Neill. Through slitted eyes I saw her short figure walking beside me. 'Put her in here.' She sounded annoyed. They lifted me on to a table. My hands moved to my throat, but she held them down. 'Just two cuts. Not deep. Give me some gauze and tape.' The swab of antiseptic stung and the adhesive across my neck was uncomfortable. 'O.K.

4

Get up, Judith. You're all right.' And she walked out of the room.

They lifted me to a sitting position. I stared at my dangling legs, ashamed to lift my eyes. Not one of them said anything to me or asked me why I had done it. For once I was glad of the apparent callousness in the ward routine. They helped me back to the Day Room and sat me down at a table. I sank my head on my chest and saw spots of blood drying brown on my dress. I wanted to cry but couldn't. I felt as I had that night at home, pleading with Jay to excite me. I felt sucked dry.

Miss Willems touched my hand. 'Why did you do it, honey? You're such a nice girl. You don't want to do anything like that.'

So I'm a nice girl. Because you're nice you can't be sick?

She squeezed my hand. My bitterness dissolved. I wanted to rush to her and loose the flood of terror in her arms. But the shame was too strong. I fingered the bandage on my neck and turned my head away.

An hour later I was called to the conference room where the nurse Mrs. Matthews had given me some cigarettes. Doctor Manning was waiting. He had his chair tilted to the wall and his long legs rested against the table. He started to talk, but I had sunk into a semi-stupor, with my head down and my hands clasped in my lap. Then I heard him say, '. . . take away your glasses.'

'Oh, no. Don't do that, please!' I jumped from my seat. 'I won't do it again. I promise. I need my glasses. I can't see without them. Please, Doctor Manning, I didn't mean it. I was just trying to show how terrible I feel.' I ripped the bandage from my neck. 'See? I hardly hurt myself. I won't do it again. I won't do anything like that. I promise. Please!' As I pleaded with him I thought, he thinks I'm crazy. A woman tries suicide twice and then insists she'd never use her glasses as a weapon because she's very near-sighted. I waited for him to laugh, but he was silent, his eyes slightly squinted.

'I'll let you have them. For a while, anyway. But you're going to be closely watched. If you try anything, I'll have to——'

The rest of his words were lost in the welter of my relief.

I walked out to the Day Room again. The patients had just returned from the cafeteria. I expected them to crowd round me with awed and anxious faces, as school children do when a pupil comes from the principal's office. But no one approached me. They picked up books, shuffled decks of cards, fingered jigsaw puzzles.

My torpor had vanished and I grew angry. 'What's the matter with you?' I cried out inside. 'Don't you want to know what happened? Why I did it? What he said to me? I could be dead by now. Why don't you care? Doesn't anybody care?'

It was *Monday, July 31st.* I was still sleeping in the utility room. Mrs. Hendricks bustled in, warm and motherly, as she had that first morning.

'Come on, honey. Got to get you up and out. Roll call soon. And breakfast. I bet you eat a good breakfast today.' She plumped the pillow in a completely unnecessary gesture; it was made of hard rubber and the head of a giant couldn't dent it.

'No, I'm not hungry, Mrs. Hendricks. What time is it?'

'Ten to six, dear.'

'But breakfast isn't until seven.'

'We have to get you up and out into the Day Room. It's Monday.'

I stared at her blankly.

'We have to get the girls ready for insulin shock. They use those two wards right off this hall.'

'It's only ten to six', I repeated, dully.

'They have to start early, honey. Are you ready?'

My stomach turned. 'Me? Am I going in there?'

'No. And don't be so scared. It's nothing bad. They're getting better. Now go on across the Day Room. Get your soap and towel from your cabinet and have a wash. Got to get this room straightened up.'

'Do they use this room for insulin shock?'

'No. This is just an extra room for sleeping when the wards are crowded.' She peered through the barred window. 'Mmn, Going to be another fine day. Now shoo. Shoo!' She prodded me good-naturedly.

'But my clothes are in there.' I pointed to the knotted sheet under the bed.

'I'll have it open by the time you get back. Now go brush your teeth, honey.'

I pattered barefoot across the Day Room, trying to keep the open-backed nightgown from flapping and shivering in the cool morning air.

I didn't have my glasses. One of the nurses had taken them when I went to bed. Where had she put them, and where was she now, and how do I get them back? Those first few days were torture. My head throbbed as I tried to remember the many faces and facets of A Ward routine. I walked around talking to myself. Who is that nurse? When did she come on? Which attendant takes care of your clothes? Whom do I ask for soap and toilet paper? What do I do when I menstruate? Order, I must have order.

The door to the big ward was open. I manoeuvred past the beds towards the row of cabinets, but without my glasses I couldn't read the names on the adhesive stickers.

'Hello, Judy.'

I turned to see Beverly, scrawny in her nightgown, the points of her flat breasts barely showing through the thin material.

'Oh, Beverly! Where's my cabinet? Do you know?'

'Next to mine. There . . . over by the dresser.'

I squinted in the direction of her finger and headed for an old walnut dressing-table with a cracked mirror on top. I spent the next half-hour shuffling from my cabinet to the crowded wash-room and back, then across the Day Room to my sleeping room.

I ran my hands down the creases of my wrinkled cotton dress. Why must we roll our clothes in bundles? Why can't we have closets and hangers?

About half a dozen women came in to crowd round the mirror in my room. I turned my head away. I have no desire to touch my face or comb my hair or look into a mirror.

'Teeth and glasses. Teeth and glasses.' A voice rang out from the corridor. A nurse was standing in the open doorway of a small utility room. I joined the patients standing in line.

'Kruger? Here.' I grabbed for my glasses and put them on my

face. The blurs and shadows disappeared. Now I knew where they put them; in a tray on a shelf in a closet in a room. Remember it.

'Come on, girls', the nurse sang out like a street pedlar. 'Last call. Teeth and glasses.'

A patient rushed up to the girl standing next to me. 'Pick up my teeth, will you? My name is Allen. I'm combing my hair in that room over there.'

There was very little I found humorous in the hospital, but this amused me. It sounded so funny. Teeth and glasses. Why not wigs and wooden legs? And trusses and hearing aids? And hearts and lungs? The same old brain this morning, girls? Why not try a fresh one? And how about a nice new heart, red and shiny and guaranteed?

Roll call, breakfast, and clean-up. Until ten o'clock in the morning, a casual observer, not knowing that this was a hospital, might watch the patients dressed in bright cotton dresses and smile. Those busy women. Sweeping and mopping and making up their beds. They look like housewives with children at school and husbands at work. Such a busy morning. But at 10 a.m. on Monday, Wednesday, and Friday, a strange machine was wheeled through the halls, across the Day Room. Then the nurses would tap certain patients on the shoulder and lead them into the big ward.

I watched and grew afraid. 'What's that?' I nudged a woman next to me.

'Electro-shock machine. You never seen one?'

'No. Are they taking those patients for shock treatment?'

'Yeah. You going?'

'No. Oh, no.'

'Judith!'

I whirled. The head nurse, Mrs. O'Neill, was standing there. 'Come. Follow me.'

'In there?' I raised a shaking hand and pointed to the main ward.

'No. Upstairs for your spinal.'

I followed her to the lift. Six other patients were waiting there with a student nurse. Their faces mirrored my own bewilderment and apprehension. After a short ride we got off and I recognized the Admissions ward where I had spent those first few hours.

'Follow me, girls', the student nurse said. She was small and blonde with a china-pink complexion.

We walked through the Admissions ward and then through another ward, the nurse unlocking and locking many doors. Then we took another lift and got off on an office floor. Small metal signs jutted out from the walls: 'Administration', 'Social Service', 'X-Ray', 'Surgery', 'Accounting', 'Dietitian'.

'Here, girls. Wait here.' The little bonde nurse poked her head into a small room and said, 'A Ward, Mr. Webber.'

A man in a white jacket was standing by a cabinet crowded with instruments. Next to him was a tall, angular nurse. The student handed a sheet of paper to her and the nurse called out the first name.

The patient walked in and the nurse closed the door. When it opened again, the student nurse had her arm round the patient.

'It hurt. It hurt', the patient said. ⁓

'But just a little bit, huh?'

'Sargent. Claire Sargent.'

When the door closed, we swarmed round the first girl.

'What did they do?' I asked.

'They stuck me with a big needle. Here.' She pointed to the base of her spine. 'This big!' She held her hands about a foot apart.

'Good God', the girl next to me whined. 'I won't let them do it.'

I was thinking. *There is no needle that big. Twenty gauge. Maybe fifteen. That's all. That's the biggest they can use. I hope.*

'Kruger. Judith.'

Remember. Be good. Don't show them it hurts. They're watching you all the time. Doctor Manning said so.

'Sit down here', the nurse said. 'Now pull up your dress from the back. Higher. Hold it. Bend over. More. More!' She leaned on me with a cold strong hand, pressing my chest against my thighs. I craned my neck to watch the man fit a needle into a syringe.

Twenty gauge. That's it. I was right. Not so big. But big enough.

The nurse pressed down again. Cold alcohol chilled my skin.

'Hold still, now.' There was a sudden, sharp, pushing pain. Then a giving way. Now a drawing out. Heavy pulling. More pain now. I gritted my teeth. Out! A quick cotton dab.

'O.K. Get up.' I felt light-headed and dizzy. The student nurse helped me out into the hall.

I had had a spinal tap, a routine test in all mental institutions. The fluid is analysed for any alteration in its normal components to rule out the possibility of organic disease such as syphilis, brain tumour, multiple sclerosis, acute infections, T.B., and meningitis, all of which may cause mental disturbance.

Every new patient had a spinal tap and every one hated it. The temporary fluid loss frequently caused headaches lasting from a few hours to several days.

I had no ill effects, but many of the patients complained of headaches. The more sympathetic nurses and attendants allowed them to rest on the beds, but when the head nurse was around they swept through the wards like a corps of M.P.'s, rapping the bed rails, pulling the patients off the beds, and herding them out to the Day Room.

It was now two in the afternoon. I was sitting on a bed in the far corner of the large sleeping ward, staring out of the window. A summer storm was brewing. The ivy leaves shivered in the wind and rustled against the outside bars. The sky was black with thunderclouds.

Suddenly I remembered the dream I had had a few nights after I returned to the apartment from the Philadelphia hospital. The baby and I were in the middle of a huge glassed-in house. It was storming and the rain seemed all round us. Then a knock on the glass door and the terrible figure of a bearded man. As soon as I saw him I knew he was a murderer. He was trying to break in the door with his fists. And then my brother was standing next to me. He opened the door and I did nothing to stop him. I was powerless with fear. The man pushed past us and ran to the white bassinet. He reached for Gary, choking, squeezing, mutilating. He killed the baby. The tiny baby. And I had done nothing to stop it. My baby was dead. But I didn't do it. It was the stranger. The crazed one. The madman. . . .

'All right. Off the bed. Come on . . . into the Day Room now.'

Miss Willems came on duty at three o'clock. She smiled at me as she walked past, and I managed a weak smile in return. 'Hello, Judy. How are you?'

'The same. No better.'

'You look better, honey. You really do. And you're going to get well. I know it.' She had a starched handkerchief in her breast pocket and it smelt of her cologne.

They all know it. So sure. So smart. See in the future, don't they? Did they know I'd tried to kill myself again? Wonder if they cleared away the glass. They were careless. Unprepared. Have to watch out for people like me. Never know what we'll do next. We're sick, but we're smart. And only we know how we feel. She means well. They all do. But were they ever sick like this? How long can a person live in fear?

The storm broke as we went to supper. By the time we came back to the Day Room the sun was out again. Long hours stretched ahead.

I moved from one table to the other, bombarding the women with questions about hospital routine. Why do we eat at four o'clock? Do you have the same bed every night? Is that a state dress you're wearing? How long have you been here?

When I sensed annoyance I moved to another spot and queried someone else. I avoided the sullen brown-haired girl who worked jigsaw puzzles all day, and when the big Hunter woman walked past the tables I stood frozen, afraid to draw her attention.

A plump, round-faced girl was playing cards. I heard her laugh a lot and her voice carried across the Day Room. Two student nurses were with her. The fourth member of the group was a thin woman with glasses. I sat down next to them. The fat girl smiled. I introduced myself.

'I'm Bertha', she said. 'And this is Laura.' She pointed to the one with glasses. I recognized the blonde nurse as the one who had taken us for our spinals that morning. The other nurse was named Nancy Mitchell.

'Bertha and I are both from Pittsburgh', Nancy said. 'I'm from St. Mary's Nursing School. We spend six weeks here as part of our training. Have you met all the girls here?'

'Which ones?' I asked.

'Us!' Bertha said, waving her arms. 'All us chickens. "Nobody here but us chickens!" ' She laughed as she scooped up the pack of cards and shuffled them expertly. 'You play bridge?' she asked.

'No. I'm not very good at cards.'

'Come on. We'll teach you. If you don't play cards you'll go crazy.' She roared at her own joke and slapped her hand on the table.

We all sat talking and playing for almost an hour. In the weeks that followed I was persuaded to try many card games: poker, pinochle, bridge . . . They had to reindoctrinate me each day in the rules of the games because my span of attention was so short.

Bertha and Laura, along with Beverly, were my closest attachments at the hospital. Laura, who was a schoolteacher, was on insulin shock. When I met her, she had received almost twenty treatments. Other than telling me her occupation, that she was unmarried, and lived with her mother, she didn't reveal much of herself or her illness. Bertha told me privately one day that when Laura was admitted she had done nothing but kneel in a corner and pray. What did she pray for, I wondered. Expiation of some inner guilt? Peace for a tortured soul? That I could use. Peace.

Laura's quiet manner was in sharp contrast to Bertha's loud and jocular personality. Bertha showed me a picture of herself, cracked and dog-eared from handling. Almost every patient who was well enough to think of home and family carried a wallet and a celluloid folder stuffed with pictures. I saw snapshots of husbands and children, babies in carriages, children on bicycles or playing in the snow. Each picture was a bridge to the past and all that came before the commitment papers had crackled stiffly in the hands of doctors, before the hurried words of explanation to children, before the wail of ambulances, or the quiet, toneless words of good-bye.

Looking at her picture and observing Bertha's behaviour, I wondered what was wrong with her. She was sociable and friendly and very lucid in her conversation with me. She never lashed out in sudden anger or lapsed into dull depressions. Her clothes were clean and neat and she took pains with her hair, her make-up, and her nails. She was on electro-shock treatment, complaining neither more nor less than the other patients. The student nurses and the rest of the staff liked her, and she co-operated willingly in the daily clean-ups. We grew close as we played cards every day, and she told me that she had a husband in the service and a young daughter living with her mother.

The only odd thing about Bertha was that she seemed happy in the hospital. But I told myself that this was impossible. No one could be happy here. If you smiled and laughed as Bertha did, it had to be a false front. Yet I admired her, envied her, and was also jealous. Whatever was wrong with her, it couldn't be serious. After all, didn't she sleep at night?

August 8

Today I started a diary. I have to pull together the fragments of this unreal existence. I have to account for it or else I will never understand it. Living is not enough.

August 9

They came as I lay in bed at night, fully clothed. It was still early. I could hear the television set blasting from the Day Room. When they turned it off I still couldn't sleep. When did I sleep last? The night before the baby came? Two months ago.

Suddenly they walked in wheeling that shock machine, and a student nurse, Bertha's friend Nancy, came to the bed and started to undress me.

'What are you doing?' I tried to sit up, but another nurse slipped off my glasses and gently pushed me back.

'We're going to make you feel better, Judith', Nancy said.

Panic closed in but it was fear of something specific, some immediate danger.

'Please don't. Give me my clothes, please!'

The rolled me to one side and slipped my arms through the sleeves of a nightgown. It smelt freshly laundered.

'That's not my nightgown. What are you going to do?' I sat up and squinted at the large white machine.

'Now lie down, Judith.' Another nurse spoke from the foot of the bed. Then Nancy reached down into a large wooden barrel and brought out rolls of wide flat rope and began to wrap them round my ankles and wrists, with the bulk of the roll hanging free over the bed. Then she ran her hands through my hair. 'Do you have any hair grips in your hair? Oh, yes. Here's two. Do you have false teeth? A plate?'

'No. But——' The terror was mounting.

'All right. That's all.'

The other nurse looked out into the corridor. 'He's not here yet.'

'Please. What's going to happen? Are you going to give me shock?' I turned from one blurry face to another.

'Now stop worrying. Lie down and relax.'

'I can't relax. Can I have a drink of water?'

'Yes. Go and get it. But hurry back.'

When I stood up the long restraints lay on the floor. 'Like this?'

'It's all right. Go ahead.'

The water from the fountain in the hall tasted warm and metallic. I spat it out.

I'm going to throw up. Can I run some place? Hide from them? These things on my feet. Scared. Scared stiff.

I went back to the room.

'Here he comes. Now get in bed, Judith.'

A tall man with yellow hair walked into the room.

'Ready, Doctor Connor.'

I strained to get up. They held my wrists and pushed me back. I couldn't see him now. He was some place behind that machine. Then he pressed something cold and wet to each of my temples.

Nancy moved next to me, her skirt billowing against my face. I stared at tiny blue and white checks.

'Open your mouth, Judith.' They pressed a tongue depressor across my teeth and tilted my head back, back, until my neck ached with the strain.

'Now hold it!'

A click and a whir came from the machine. And I heard his voice say, 'Shock!'

Was it an instant or time without measure? . . .

I came to consciousness standing up. My bare feet were on a cold, wet floor and I was tired, so terribly tired, and dripping with perspiration. Then I felt water rushing over me. Someone was lifting my arms and turning me round and round. The water beat against my face. Then it stopped. Someone was shaking me and calling, Judith! Judith!

A name. Whose name? Mine? I couldn't remember who I was or where I was or what had happened. My head throbbed as I tried to orient myself. I knew no past or present. My memory had disappeared.

I clutched the hand of this woman. 'Where . . .?' My voice was cracked and hoarse.

'You're in the shower, Judith. You just had a shock treatment and now you're in the shower.' I looked around cautiously. 'You'll get your bearings in a few minutes and you'll be all right.'

Bearings? (*North, east, south, west. Home is best. What home? And what is my last name and where am I?*) Tears sprang to my eyes. (*So tired. Want to lie down and cry and never stop crying.*) She held a towel out for me. I couldn't lift my arms to take it.

'Who are you?'

'Nancy Mitchell. Remember?'

She rubbed me dry and dressed me in a nightgown. 'All right, Judith. This way. Across the hall. Back to your room.'

I looked at the strange surroundings and fear snaked through my body. I grabbed both her hands. 'Please. Where am I?'

She smiled and squeezed my hands a little. 'State Hospital. Ward A. Now get into bed and rest. I'll come back to see you soon.'

As soon as she left I jumped up. Her skirt. Blue and white checks. I've seen it before. Where, where, where . . . Suddenly the mind vacuum filled and I knew. I'm Judith Kruger. I have a husband Jay. My baby is Gary. I paced up and down the room. Who's with him? Oh, yes—my mother. She's at home. In . . . in . . . Philadelphia. I dropped to my knees, pressed my palms against the floor, and wept.

But how long ago . . . did they turn on a machine . . . did a man in a brown suit say 'shock'? There's a clock somewhere. I remember a clock. I rushed into the hall and peered up. There it is. Big clock. Big

*hands. I can read it. It says 9.30. No. 8.30. a.m.? or p.m.? What day
is it? Have to know how long.*

Light streamed from the nursing office. I know that nurse.
Mrs. Matthews. Gave me cigarettes. Nice woman.

'Mrs. Matthews. I had a treatment. A shock treatment.'

'I know. How do you feel?'

'I forgot everything.'

'It'll all come back to you. Now go to sleep.'

'What day is it, please?'

'The same day. Eight-thirty.'

And I remembered looking at the clock when I went for some
water. It had read 10 minutes to 8. Could it possibly be? Only
forty minutes ago?

'Are you sure?'

She smiled a little. 'I'm sure. You have to sleep now. Don't
you feel tired?'

'Yes. I feel tired. Thank you.'

I went back to the room and lay on the bed. Forty minutes.
A short eternity. What is it they do to strip a mind so fast?
Electric shock. A shock with electricity. Why? To make me
better? Don't feel better. Just so tired. Exhausted. Every
muscle . . . every nerve . . . my legs . . . and arms . . . and
eyes . . . so tired . . .

I woke up this morning at six-thirty. For the first time in
eight weeks I had slept. For ten hours. Without sedation. And
there was peace. And calm. And a quiet inside me.

Wednesday afternoon, August 9

Another shock treatment in the morning. But this time I
knew what was coming, and some of the fear was diluted and
diverted into hate, a specific hate for the entire procedure.
Now that I know what to expect I can handle it. It's the
massive non-directed fear of my sickness that makes me so
helpless.

I didn't fight them or complain. I did everything they told
me to do. The same doctor was there, and again he didn't say
a word. Would it have killed him to say a word of comfort?
Do they think it's easy, this submission to oblivion? Wonder
how the other patients take it?

. . . Came to in the shower again. The same amnesia. The same wasteland of forgetting. But this time I waited for memory and orientation to return. I told myself if not this minute, then the next, or the next. And again the aching all over my body. What happens when I'm in shock? Do I struggle? I must ask Jay when he comes this Sunday.

I lay on my bed all afternoon. But they kept rousing me, shoving me out to the Day Room.

Why the hell can't they leave me alone?

Thursday, August 10

Nancy Mitchell told me that electro-shock is administered only three times a week because daily treatments would cause too much confusion and memory loss. I like Nancy and the other student nurses. They're young. And friendly. They talk to us and tell us things. I'm afraid of the older nurses. You can't ask them any questions. They cut you short. They're always rushing in and out of the office. They act as though we're in the way. Don't they know if it weren't for us they wouldn't have a job?

They put Helen Jacoby in the solitary room this morning. She's so pretty, with that yellow hair and blue eyes. And so sweet. She has two little boys. I saw their picture. I wonder what happened to her? She came a week before I did and is also on shock. She was doing so well. One minute she was fine, sitting with us in the Day Room and talking and laughing. Then she walked away, into the big ward. Some of the girls who saw her said she started to undress herself and tore her clothes and mumbled and cried.

When we lined up for cafeteria we passed the row of isolation rooms. Beverly was behind me.

'They put Helen there', she whispered. 'There. That room.'

I didn't want to look. See no sickness, hear no sickness, feel no sickness. Like a superstition. Make believe it didn't happen, that they are just acting.

But I did look. I stood on tiptoe and peered through the bars. Padded walls. A small wooden cot. No pillows. No chairs. Where was she? The window! She had climbed up and was clinging to the top window bars.

I cried out inside. Helen. Helen. Don't hang there like an animal, please. It hurts me and frightens me. Helen, you're so nice. Please get down. Say something like, oh, pardon me, I didn't know you were there.. I was just looking out of the window. It's a lovely day. Wait a minute. I'm coming. I'll be right with you, girls.

'Keep moving, A Ward. Keep moving.' The attendant's voice was loud behind me. 'Cafeteria, girls. Let's go. *Let's go!*'

Nobody here talks much about a disturbed patient. They seem to ignore the fact that a bridge partner doesn't come back to finish her hand or that the girl in the next bed was taken away in the night. Do they feel the way I did when I looked at Helen? Or maybe they just don't care. Like stones in a raging river, they are unmoved by the human tide churning round them.

Friday, August 11th

One small pleasure I enjoy is smoking in the washroom after breakfast. It's almost like a social hour. We talk and smoke until clean-up is over. Still have no desire to help. Wonder if they have a book, a black-list, with the names of the women who rush to the washrooms to smoke instead of helping to clean the wards? Doctor Manning said they'd watch me. Can they find me in there? Do they miss me outside? Oh, to hell with it!

Beverly sat with me in the Day Room. Showed me another letter from her brother. She carries them round like love letters. She must be crazy about him. I can't talk to her for too long. Something about her eyes and the way she slumps when she walks.

At nine-thirty the head nurse tapped me on the shoulder. 'Get undressed, Judith.' I started to ask her why, but she was walking away. I ran after her.

'Mrs. O'Neill. Why must I get undressed now?'

'You're on shock with the rest of them this morning. Go into the main ward. In the bathroom.'

There were about fifteen women there when I walked in. They were stripping themselves, rolling up their clothes, and laying the bundles on the floor in neat little rows. A student nurse gave each of them a name stick and a clean nightgown.

Undress and dress, dress and undress. Pain in the neck routine.
When I get out of here I'll sleep in my clothes.

The washroom seemed strange. No smoke, no talk, no
laughter. When I came out into the ward it was cleared of
loiterers and the door to the Day Room was closed. I saw the
large wooden barrels and I knew that they held the rolls of
restraints. Student nurses were stripping the beds down to the
red rubber mattresses and making them up again with two sets
of sheets. Little cardboard tags were tied to the footrails.
They looked like the kind that railway porters attach to out-
going baggage. I still had my glasses and I walked past the beds
checking names. Mine was the sixth bed. The tag was new and
the ink was fresh. I went back to the washroom. It was more
crowded now. Beverly was there. And Bertha. And Esther, the
blonde grandmother. She was wriggling into her nightgown
and fumbling with the button at the back.

'Well, here we go again, girls! Another day, another shock.
Nothing like a good shock to start off the day.' Some of the
women giggled, but their eyes weren't laughing.

Mrs. O'Neill poked her head in at the door. 'All those with
glasses and false teeth give them to me. And everybody get in
their beds.'

'O.K., girls. Out with the teeth. Spit 'em out!' Esther talked
under her breath. 'And the goggles. And the wooden legs.
Hearing aids. Bust pads. Oh, everything . . . I have . . . is
yours', she hummed. This time we laughed outright.

She's got guts, I thought. How long does it take before you
can joke about shock?

I lay on my bed. Aimless, restless half-thoughts skirted round
the core of fear.

They rolled the big barrel to my bed and wrapped my wrists
and ankles with restraints. Then I sat up and squinted down the
line of beds. Most of the women were lying down. I heard no
sound of crying.

Good girls. We're all good little girls.

The door creaked open and they wheeled in the shock
machine. Then they set up a portable hospital screen between
the first two beds. I wondered how the first girl felt. Is it better
to be the first to go? Sounds like death. I flung my hands back

and gripped the cold metal bed frame. Then the sweat came and the urge to urinate and the shrivelling in the bowels and the thick furriness in the mouth.

I heard the machine squeak as they rolled it and then the voice of the doctor. 'Shock!'

My body tensed, and I waited for the scream. But it wasn't a scream or a cry or a moan. It was an animal sound from a human throat. A grunting and a rasping. Like a death rattle, rising, then falling away. I raised myself up and saw the screen move with a squeal of casters. Again the sharp command and the unnatural sound.

Coming closer. Closer to me. I yelled at them with my lips shut tight—*Why must I watch and wait and hear them cry out?*

Then they were next to me. I know what's coming and the knowing is worse than not knowing. It shouldn't be, but it is. It is. . . . Wood against my teeth, hands pushing on my head, wetness by the ears. Any minute, any second now. Tell them you hate——

'Shock!'

Saturday, August 12

There's a new patient in the ward. Her name is Mary. She's only sixteen years old and I think she's a prostitute. She talked to me in the Day Room this morning.

'Hello. I'm Mary. What's your name?'

I looked up into a pale, pretty face, a little pinched and tight round the nose and ears. She was tall and thin and had long brown hair pulled back from her ears with a dirty ribbon. A thick smear of lipstick covered her small mouth.

'I'm Judith Kruger', I answered.

'I just came from the ward upstairs. I liked it. I like it here, too. The girls are nice. Do you like me, Judith?'

'Why yes. Sure I do.'

'Do I look all right? They gave me this dress but it don't have much style. I'm trying to fix it so I'll look good.'

She was wearing a faded state dress. I had on a state dress, too. I had told the attendants that my mother was too busy caring for my baby to wash and iron my clothes. It was a lie. I had many dresses in my bin in the storage closets. But I didn't want to touch or feel anything that was mine. Fear of things put me here, I told myself. Too many things. Blankets and dresses and nappies and shoes and moving and packing. New things. Old things. Everything. If I could have walked round naked I would have done so.

'Well, tell me. Does it look good?'

She had pulled the belt in tight round her waist and hiked up the skirt under the belt so that the dress came above her knees. The half sleeves were rolled up over the curve of her shoulder and the neckline was tucked in around and under her brassière straps. She had tried to fashion the housedress into a sarong.

'Don't you have it a little too tight?'

'Oh, no. I like it that way. It looks sexy.'

I couldn't prevent my next question. 'Why do you want to look sexy?'

'So men will want me.'

It was a wrong thing to do, but I couldn't help it. I laughed.

'Men? Here? You're in a hospital, Mary.'

'They have doctors here, don't they?'

'Do you think they'll notice you? I mean, have time for that sort of thing? This is a busy place.'

'I know. Want to know something? I like it here. It's like home, but better. I been in lots of places. Welfare places. Once I was in a home for delinquent girls. They said I stole a lady's pocketbook, but I didn't. It was mine. I bought it. They were mean to me. They're nice here. Like a big family.'

'Don't you have parents?'

'They're separated. I don't know. Anyway, I ran away.'

'What did you do?'

'Sleep with men.' Her eyes were frank and open and there was no shame in her voice.

'Are you serious, Mary? How old are you? Sixteen?'

'I had a boy friend twenty-eight.'

'You had sex relations with men?'

'Plenty of times. Why not? I got to go now. I want to set my hair. Do you think I should wear it up for tonight?' With a surprisingly graceful gesture, she lifted both hands and lifted her hair high on her head.

'What's tonight?'

'Nothing. I just like to look pretty at night.' She walked through the Day Room, her little buttocks bouncing under the tight skirt.

A kid. Just a baby. She's sick. And I fell for her talk. And yet . . . I'm twenty-eight and I feel like a child.

I saw her again after lunch. It was hot in the Day Room. I put my head down on the table but lifted it quickly. I knew I mustn't let them think I was sluggish or lazy or uninterested in my surroundings. They're watching me even when they walk hurriedly through the wards on their way from someplace to somewhere. . . .

'No! No! No! Mrs. O'Neill. It's mine! It's mine!'

Mary was running through the Day Room, yelling after the head nurse. Tears streaked the heavy powder on her face. Hair grips were sticking from the torn kerchief wrapped round her head.

'Mary, I told you it's not yours. You can't have it. Now go sit down.'

'I tell you it's mine! That talcum powder is mine. It's a green box with silver letters. It's mine.'

'It was in your cabinet, but it doesn't belong to you. We put adhesive stickers on all patients' articles. See here. On the bottom. Helene Robbins. That's the girl next to you. You took it.'

'It's a lie!' Her voice was desperate and ugly. 'You're making it up. It belongs to me. I hate you! Hate you', she screamed at the nurse's disappearing back. She stamped her feet and balled her hands into fists. Now she really looked like a child.

Nobody spoke to her. She turned to me and grabbed my shoulder, digging her nails into my flesh.

'Tell her I didn't take it. Tell that nurse. She hates me.'

I pried her fingers loose. 'I thought you said you liked this place.' I was taking a sudden sadistic pleasure in torturing her. (*Smug little thing. Sleeps with men, does she?*) 'You told me that this morning, didn't you?'

Her body sagged, and she sniffled. 'I do like it. All except her. She doesn't let you have anything. There's a bitch upstairs the same way. Took away my magazine. I wrote my name on it but she kept saying I took it off another girl. They don't let you have nothing around here.'

She wiped away the tears with the back of her hand and stalked out of the Day Room, kicking over a chair.

. Laura and Bertha had been standing by the door to the big ward. Now they came over to me.

'She steals things', Laura said, her dark eyes tinged with pity. 'She took one of little Nancy's colouring books yesterday . . . you know how she leaves things all over the Day Room. She's such a sick child, Judith. I feel so sorry for her.'

'I do too', I echoed.

Unconsciously we both turned to Bertha, expecting a like answer. For an instant I thought her fat face looked scared. 'Cards, Laura? Judith?' Then she smiled in her usual way. 'Tennis, anyone?' Her laugh echoed through the Day Room.

Sunday, August 13

Today was visiting day. My father came. I was one of the first to be called. I was standing near the telephone in the main ward and when the nurse picked up the phone she nodded at me.

'O.K., Judith. Your father. Go ahead.'

He was stepping off the lift as I ran through the Day Room. The sun hit his glasses and made a yellow spotlight on his face. He looked so old and tired that I wanted to cry. I ran to him, talking to myself.

Daddy. Daddy. It hurts me. To see you and to have you come and see me. I know you're sad and worried and you can't believe I'm here. You don't know what happened to your daughter and neither do I, Daddy. Neither do I.

'Hello, Dad.' I reached him and touched his hand as he bent to kiss me.

'Hello, darling', he said. There were tears in his eyes.

Don't, Daddy, please. Don't cry for me. I'm not worth it. Quickly, now. Talk . . . start talking.

'How's Mother?'

'Fine. Everything's fine.'

'Jay's on duty at the hospital, isn't he? He wrote me last week he'd be on duty.'

'Yes. He sends his love and said thanks for his birthday card. It came the day after. He showed it to us.'

'I made it myself. I couldn't buy a card here.'

'It was lovely, darling.'

'Oh, yes. Lovely. (*Cardboard end sheet from my writing-pad. Folded in quarters. Punched through with a pencil. Little love words. Guilt words.*) Nice birthday time for him, huh?'

'It's all right, darling. It's all right.' He patted my hand. 'Everything will be all right.'

'You took the bus here, Dad?'

'Yes.'

'You didn't have to. I mean, it's so early to get a bus just to get here by nine. Just for two hours.'

'So what?' He tried to be brusque and jocular at the same time. 'Do you think I'd miss seeing you?'

I remembered visiting Sundays when I was ten, at summer camp. I never had to wonder whether they would come. They always did, were always there, with all the little things I had asked for. They never disappointed me.

He began to fumble with a big package. 'Fruit and cake and cookies. O.K.?'

'Sure, Dad. Fine. Fine.'

'And here's the knitting bag you asked for in your letter. Is it all right? Mother got it at a five-and-ten up the street.'

I tried to visualize the streets around our home in Philadelphia. I had lived there for only eight days.

'Fine! Just what I want. I can carry my cigarettes—we're not supposed to smoke, but we do. I get them from other girls. And a nice nurse gives me a packet sometimes. Dad, next time would you bring more cigarettes? I can carry them in this bag. Tell Mom thanks.'

'What dress are you wearing, Judy? That's not one of yours, is it?'

'No. It's a state dress. I don't want to use up my clothes. You'd have to take them home when they're dirty and Mother has no time to wash and iron.'

'Isn't that silly? You have plenty of clothes. Why wear——'

'It's not silly. Please. You don't understand. Don't question me, please, Dad.'

'All right. All right.' His face fell and then brightened. 'You didn't ask about the baby.'

'Oh, yes. Sure. How is he?' I really didn't want to know.

'Fine. Wonderful. A doll. Just a doll. He's adorable. If you could see him. So tiny. Like this.' He made a little cupping gesture with his hands and chuckled the way he always did about babies. 'And you know what?' He pulled his chair close to me and held my hands. 'He's beginning to look for his thumb. Oh, is that cute! He tries all round his face but misses his mouth. Like this. See?'

'Dad, please. Somebody will see you. I mean, you look so funny. (*Silly-funny. Always embarrassed when he acts so kittenish. Now say something to take the sting away.*) I feel a little better, Dad.'

'You look better.'

'I was very depressed. The first days here were terrible.'

'But you're better now?'

'I'm getting electro-shock treatments. Did you know?'

'Well, Jay, he——'

'Do you know what they're like? I hate them. They make you unconscious and you have a convulsion and——'

He cut me off. 'The main thing is that you're better.'

I knew it. He doesn't want to hear about it. Doesn't want to hear the ugly parts.

'I've had three so far.'

'Mother will be glad to hear you're better.'

Afraid to listen to me, Dad? Afraid to find out what they're doing to your little girl?

Something evil prodded me on. I insisted on telling him of all the strangeness here . . . the real crazy ones, the screams, the terror, and the fear. I sucked out his pity the way I've always done with Dad and Mother, and then refused his concern with a show of bravado and resignation . . . What's wrong with me?

Gloria had visitors this morning, too. She told me she saw me with my father and that I looked just like him. I've always felt uncomfortable when people tell me that, as though I must defend myself or make some sort of excuse.

Gloria was in the Admissions ward the night I came. I didn't see her again until a few days ago when they brought her down to A Ward, but I remembered her face. Long and thin and pockmarked. Pretty grey eyes. Waving brown hair.

We talked for a little while after cafeteria.

'You know, Judy,' she said, 'we all thought you had pull to get out of Admission so quickly and get down here.'

'What do you mean, "we"?'

'Oh, all the girls up there. We figured it was because your husband was a doctor.'

'Oh, no. Not that at all. It didn't have anything to do with my husband. (*Why do they think that? I don't have pull. I don't deserve it. And I don't want them to talk about me and my husband and point fingers and stare when I'm not looking. Not here. Not in this place.*) What's wrong with you, Gloria?'

'My stomach. Pains. Like rumblings and cramps. I can't hold much food down. Maybe it's my gall bladder. I eat with the insulin patients. They get a special non-fat diet. And they're giving me tests. Metabolism. Things like that.'

'That's all?'

'What do you mean? Isn't that enough? Those pains are awful.'

'Are you nervous or afraid, like me?'

No pride or discretion. Let them all know that I'm sick.

'No, I'm not nervous. But I get terrible headaches. And I can't gain weight.'

'Oh. Well, maybe you'll get better here, Gloria.'

'I hope so.' She walked away and I stared after her.

There's something she didn't tell me. There must be something else. Stomach trouble and headaches and for that she lets them put her in a mental hospital, huh? I don't believe her.

Don't know whom to believe. No line between the real and the unreal here, between actuality and sick imagination.

Monday, August 14

Had the fourth bed in the row for my fourth shock. Not so bad this time. Less waiting, less fear. Have begun to realize all the levels of fear a person can experience.

Tension. The burning eyes and tightness in the neck. Clammy

hands and perspiration. Tension is trying. To grasp something new and conquer it. To produce and succeed. Tension lives in the muscles and the brain.

Worry. I know how to worry. It's easy. I worry very well in bed. Lie there and let a thousand prickly thoughts wash over you like waves. One after another. Something you did wrong or said wrong. Something to come that will test you. Anticipation and recapitulation.

Real Fear. I know what that is, too. Afraid of being hurt. That's when your heart pounds and your bowels loosen. You want to run but the feet are leaden. The power drains out of you and you can't move or think.

These I understand. But the fear I've been living with for the past two months is so totally different. It's all-inclusive, all-encompassing. It hovers and smothers and chokes. I can't find the right words for this fear. It's not a segment of my existence, it's the whole of me. Yet I continue to exist. I have no delusions, no hallucinations. But I walk and talk and breathe with fear. Like a thing alive, too big to fight, too heavy to push away.

Night-time now. I'm in my bed in the main ward. They transferred me here a few days ago. It's not bad. I sleep fitfully, but it's not the other patients' fault. So far no screaming here. Some of them act as though they were living in a happy place like a boarding school or a summer camp. They visit at each other's beds, and sit with scrubbed faces and hair in curlers, exchanging magazines. I can't be like that. Not for a moment do I forget that I am an inmate here. I must get out. I've got to get well and get out.

Tuesday, August 15

Tuesdays and Thursdays are good days. I can get dressed in the morning knowing I won't have to undress again and then hunt down my clothes bundle in the fog of post-shock forgetting.

There's an old upright piano in the main ward. I heard it play today. Many of the keys are dead, the foot pedals don't work, and it has a tinny sound. A patient I don't know came over to the bench and sat down. She opened a frayed hymn-book, played one selection, and left.

I slithered on to the bench and riffled through the sheet music scattered on the top, trying to look casual, but I was very excited inside. I opened the music to 'Over the Rainbow' and picked out the melody. My hands were shaking as they had done when I tried to work that girl's jigsaw puzzle. But it wasn't from fear this time. I shook with joy, the way a cripple does when he takes those first wavering steps on his own. When I finished I looked at my hands resting on the keys. They didn't look like my hands. They looked strong.

All afternoon I thought of what I had accomplished. To be able to concentrate on a specific task, and to think of birds flying over the rainbow and why oh why can't I? To experience a feeling other than fear.

Mustn't get too optimistic over this. Tomorrow I'll probably feel lousy again.

There's another patient here who plays an instrument, and very well. I heard her before I saw her. After supper the ward was almost empty. Almost everyone was in the washroom or in the Day Room. I was counting the sheets in my writing pad and had just closed the door to my cabinet when the sudden sound of music broke the stillness.

I saw no one. At first I thought it came from the television set in the Day Room, but the music was too loud and close. I stood up and looked round. In a far corner on the last bed was a figure of a woman huddled over an accordion, her body seeming to caress it. She didn't look up when I walked over. The instrument was new and the silver stops glinted under the unshaded electric light. She was playing something loud—some sort of march.

She was a big woman, wide-hipped and heavy in the legs. Her feet were planted square on the floor and the fat rippled along the back of her arms as she pumped in and out. Her face was broad, with dark, overhanging brows.

When she stopped I said, 'You play very well.' No answer.

She shifted the accordion higher on her chest and fingered the keys idly, tilting her head to catch the soft, muted notes. Suddenly, without looking at me, she said, 'My name is Florence Adamski. What's yours?'

'Judith Kruger. You play beautifully, Florence.'

'Thanks.' She still didn't look at me. 'This is the baby.' She slapped the accordion and then ran her stubby fingers over the keys in a loud arpeggio.

'You like music?'

'Oh, yes. Very much.'

'I love it. It's different from anything else. Music isn't mean.' Her voice was rough, almost like a man's.

She lifted her head. The pale grey eyes, almost without colour, were startling in her heavy face. She shifted her position on the bed and the springs squealed. I thought she would continue to play, but her fingers didn't move. She kept staring at me or through me—I couldn't tell which. I felt uncomfortable.

'Uh, are you married, Florence?'

'Yes. I got two boys. Regular Indians. That's the way I like them.'

'Does your husband play, too?'

She gripped the handles and her knuckles went white. 'My husband can go to hell. Straight to hell.'

'I'm sorry', I stammered. 'I didn't mean——'

'Don't be sorry. You don't know my husband. Haw! That's funny.' She threw back her head and laughed. 'Tonight I'm just fooling around. This is nothing. I got a whole repertoire. When I get started nothing stops me. Nothing.'

'You new here?' Two patients were standing behind me. One of them had her finger pointed at Florence.

'No. I'm old', Florence answered. 'Very old. What's your name?'

'Virginia', the woman said.

'Carry Me Back to Old Virginia. Haw! That's funny. You're old, too. Know that song? I play it good.' She began the first few bars, then stopped. 'I'm tired now, girls. Go find something to do.' Her grey eyes looked up at us blandly.

The two women turned away. I walked across the ward and didn't turn my head until I had rounded the corner of the washroom where Florence couldn't see me. Suddenly there was a wild burst of music, the notes breaking one on the other. I peeked out at her. She was hunched over the accordion, her head bobbing and weaving, and her arms working like pistons. I thought of her words, 'Music isn't mean.' Yet there was

a kind of fury in those chords crashing through the empty
ward.

Wednesday, August 16

Had my fifth shock today. Beverly told me that the usual
course of treatment is twenty. Good God! Do I have to go
through this fifteen more times? Wish I could verify this with a
doctor, but there doesn't seem to be any around. Doctor
Manning is on leave. That Doctor Connor shows up just to
administer shock and then disappears. He doesn't know me
from Adam. There are sixty patients in A Ward—more come
in each day. Feel like a pebble on a beach.

If it's not raining, they take us out on the grounds every
afternoon. I like to sit next to Miss Willems. She's so pretty and
smells so sweet and she smiles at me as if she means it. I wonder
if she knows how much I like her.

Behind the tree under which we sit is a rise of ground. A road
starts there. I can see it when the land slopes down. It stretches
so far that it must be the way out of here.

How will I feel when they release me and I walk down that
road? Will I want to go? Or will I be afraid? I don't like it here,
but it's safe. I know the routine now; where and when to eat
and sleep, to smoke, to rest, to read, to talk. No decisions to
make, no challenges to meet.

And here I don't have to look at my baby. That's the crux of
it. I barely remember what he looks like and I wish I would
never have to see him again.

Thursday, August 17

Esther is so damn funny we can't help but laugh at her and
with her. She reminds me a little of myself and how I used to be,
using exaggerated humour to ingratiate myself with strangers.
Tonight she told us she's been here for ten years and that she's
had 595 shock treatments and since she's so experienced she's
going to start giving shock to every damned doctor and nurse
in the place.

I don't know what's wrong with her, but I like her. When a
patient collars you and holds you with her eyes and tells you
how unhappy she is and asks when will she go home, you can't

do anything but mumble excuses and walk away. Esther doesn't make the rest of us uncomfortable.

I've stopped telling everybody I meet how I feel. I'm still sick, but I'm trying to keep my feelings to myself. It's hard to do. Very hard. Wish to hell there was a doctor here to talk to.

Friday, August 18

My lower lip is sore and puffed up. I bit it during the shock convulsion. Now I know why patients with false teeth have to take out their plates. They would rattle loose during the initial tremor and choke them.

Don't even care about the lip. Feel wonderful. A new doctor is now supervising A Ward while Doctor Manning is on leave. His name is Doctor Heineman. He came over to me when I was sitting in the Day Room after shock.

'Judith,' he said, 'we will give you treatment only two times in the week now. Monday and Friday.'

He walked away before I had a chance to stammer out a thank-you. But he didn't get far. Patients swarmed round him like bees. I didn't have to hear them because I knew what they were saying.

'. . . Doctor Heineman, when will I go to Staff? . . . How many more treatments will I need, Doctor? . . . Can't I go home now, Doctor? . . . Say, Doctor, can I talk with you, please? . . . They promised me a pass last week but it didn't come . . . do you know why? . . . Doctor Heineman wait! . . . just a minute, I want to know how long . . . how long . . .' Pleading, hungry faces trying to hold him with words. I saw the back of his head bob up and down like a mechanical toy as he pressed through the crowd, out into the hall, and entered the nursing office and closed the door. And I wondered how he felt as he made his escape. Was there a sense of helpless sympathy? A feeling of inadequacy? Annoyance, perhaps? Or did he feel like God?

Sunday, August 20

Jay came today and I was ashamed to see him. The first two weeks here were the same as at home. He was swallowed up in the dead emptiness of feeling and association. Now it is different. The cloud of panic has lifted. And with the lifting come shame and guilt—for having had a breakdown, for causing him trouble and worry at the beginning of his internship year ... The sight of him made me squirm.

My cheeks were burning as I walked through the ward door this morning and into the Day Room. He was walking with my father. They were both smiling.

Jay reached me first. 'Hello, sweetie.'

Why did he say that? It's no good now. Everything's changed. Don't you remember what I did with the photographs of us that you propped up on your dresser when I came home from the Philadelphia hospital? I stuck them in a drawer. Immediately. I couldn't stand them.

'Hello, Jay ... Dad. How are you?'

'Fine, fine.'

That ring in your voice. So hearty and reassuring. Are you quivering inside the way I am? This is pain for me. Shame-pain. How I wish I had written you not to come. Why can I bear Daddy's face better than yours? Why have I always been afraid of you?

Talking and talking and uneasy pauses and then more talking.

Daddy, you smile at me and humour me and make awkward little jokes. Your eyes dart and your mouth is tight and your hands move too much. You still don't know what's with me, do you? But I don't mind so terribly much. Not with you. But what do YOU feel, Jay? You're holding back, the way you always do, with that quiet control that scares me. Please don't hate me. I know you should, but please don't. I'm so ashamed. So guilty. So sick.

When he reached for my hands and tried to kiss me good-bye, I turned my face. His lips barely brushed my cheek.

Monday, August 21

Memory loss after shock today was the most severe so far. I stood in the shower naked in body and mind. I couldn't recall the date, or the baby's name, or who was with him at home.

As soon as I was dressed I ran to my cabinet and pulled out that little white card I had written on the bus ride here. My hands shook so that it was hard to read the words. Name, age, address, telephone number, our New York address, baby's name. Date and place of his birth. First names of my family. And Social Security number.

Why in hell did I put that down?

I talked to myself. Here. This is you. The people you belong to. You wrote it down for emergencies like this one. Did some strange psychic part of you suspect that this might happen? Here it is in black and white. Believe it. You have nothing else to believe. The eyes of memory are blind. Now go out into the Day Room and wait.

It took one hour of walking through corridors, talking to people with a voice in a body in a mind of no recall. Suddenly it happened just before we went to lunch. Like water rushing over a dam. I remembered everything the shock had swept away.

And then the fear crept in. Not panic-fear. This is specific. I am afraid to take care of the baby; to touch him and hold him and feed him and dress him. Could this single fear be the root? It's too simple. Too terribly simple.

Wednesday, August 23

Wednesdays are good now. No shock on Wednesdays.

Three-quarters of my waking hours are spent walking from one bathroom to the next, smoking and talking to the patients who wander in and out. I keep all my cigarettes in that knitting bag Mother sent me. Also my matches and paper hankies, toilet paper, soap, an extra towel, pencils, and notebook. I never let this bag out of my sight. I take it to cafeteria, I take it outside, and I sleep with it.

Some of them laugh at me. 'What are you carrying in there, Judy? Gold? Don't you ever put that thing down?' I don't care if they tease me. Just as long as no one puts a hand on that bag. I'd hit them if they did that.

Sometimes I think this place looks like a summer camp. But I was happy at camp, and I'm not happy here. And yet, the lawns and the trees outside, the rows of beds, the time spent in the washrooms—all are like distorted throwbacks to camp. One night during my first year as a counsellor, I remember patrolling the campus with two of my friends. Then we went into the toilet and sat on the floor. We smoked furtively and nibbled crackers and caviar from a Bronx delicatessen. We thought it uproariously funny to be eating caviar not two feet from the toilets. I was only eighteen then.

I liked camp. For two months I wore shorts and socks and played with kids. I was governed by rules. It was a safe and ordered place.

It's safe here, too. With plenty of rules and regulations. And I huddle in corners here, smoking forbidden cigarettes and trading gossip. I eat and sleep and shower and dress with hundreds of others. At camp my little cabinet was made from an orange crate. Now I have a metal one. I send and receive letters from home. And the nurses censor our mail just as the counsellors did at camp. I get packages from home. I am a name on a list in the main office. I am a face to count and my voice says 'Here' when they call the roll. They plan the days for us. At camp we always had volley ball at ten o'clock. Now it's electro-shock. Many of us were sent here by force, not so unlike a child sent away by his parents when he wants to stay in the city. Many kids endure forced holidays. We do, too. There is only one big difference here. We don't go home when summer ends.

Thursday, August 24

That fear of responsibility for the baby keeps nagging at me. I'll never manage a house and a child. It's too much. Everything is too much.

Whenever I pass the big clock in the hall I take my pulse. It's always between 90 and 110. It's stupid to keep checking like that. I know I'm nervous. My hands shake and my eyes burn and my chest and neck are knotted. Yet I must prove it by the pulse. If they gave me my watch I would take my pulse every five minutes. . . .

Something very nice happened tonight. We went to a concert. After supper Mrs. Matthews came into the Day Room. She's so short and fat her walk is like a waddle. But I like her.

She called out to us, 'Who wants to go to the Auditorium? There's a concert there tonight, girls. Line up by the nurses' office. You have ten minutes.'

I was sitting with Beverly and Bertha and Laura. We exchanged hesitant glances.

'I like music', Laura said.

'So do I', I replied. 'Bev?'

'I have to write my brother', she said. 'I didn't write him for a week. He'll worry. I know he'll worry. I want to tell him I'm not feeling so good. Do you think they'll let it pass if I say that?'

'I don't know', I answered curtly. (*She's got a chance to do something and she's thinking of her goddam brother.*) 'I'm going to line up. You coming, Laura?'

'Yes.' She turned to Bertha, who was shuffling cards aimlessly. A wad of chewing gum puffed out her plump cheeks. 'No', she said. 'I think I'll play some solitaire.'

Suddenly I was all keyed up. 'Come on, Laura. Let's not be late.'

When Mrs. Matthew checked us off there were only twenty of us. When we stepped off the lift I had no idea which building we were in. Every time I leave our ward I realize the enormity of this place. If only I could stand outside with someone to identify the buildings. I wonder how the others feel? The other thousands. Are they choking for freedom to move around, to see something beyond the walls and windows and doors of their wards? Or don't they care?

We marched along a long corridor, walked down a short flight of steps, and into a large auditorium. For an instant I thought I was back in college, walking down the balcony steps of the Auditorium.

I manœuvred to the front of the line and took the first seat in the row reserved for A Ward. Across the aisle the sections were filling up with male patients. I looked to my left and saw a young man with curly black hair and a thin, studious face. He was wearing denim trousers and a faded blue work shirt. He wore no belt or tie. He was looking straight ahead, his hands folded in his lap. He looked like a freshman student waiting for an orientation lecture.

Suddenly I quivered. Not from fear. From excitement. The kind of excitement a woman feels when she's close to a man. Any man. Am I getting well, or is this a sickness, too?

'Ladies and gentlemen. May I have your attention, please?'

A stout woman was standing on the platform. She had a rose pinned to the bosom of her dress. 'We have a very interesting programme for you this evening. Mr. and Mrs. Thomas of the

St. Christopher's Choral Group will entertain you with a variety of familiar and well-loved songs.'

She turned to a Negro couple who came out of the wings and on to the stage. They were both tall. The woman was wearing a long red gown and the man was in tails.

Soft chords from a piano rippled through the Auditorium. I craned my neck to see the pianist. As the couple stepped forward, I thought *are they afraid of us? Have they ever performed before such an audience? I wonder what they'll do if somebody screams.*

The man was a bass-baritone; the woman a mezzo-soprano. Their voices were strong and well trained and they sang with feeling and a good sense of drama: 'Summertime', 'Old Man River', 'If I Loved You', 'Kiss Me Again', and 'Smiling Through', They closed with 'Ave Maria'.

The applause, hesitant at first, grew steadily. Some of the men were cheering and whistling. I clapped until my palms were stinging and tears clouded my eyes. When I walked out through the empty rows I looked at the stage and my throat was tight with unshed tears.

Thank you. Thank you very much for coming, for looking at us, for smiling, for the music and the beauty. There is so little that is beautiful here.

Friday, August 25

Memory loss after shock is getting worse. It's like waking up from the nowhere into anywhere. Today in the shower room I burst into a fit of crying. I cried in anger and despair and resentment and helpless fury. I wanted to scream and fall down on the floor and bang the wall and yell my head off until everything they had blown to pieces grew whole again. I didn't want to wait, passive and dumb, until the hours passed and memory returned. I wanted to run through the wards and find that shock machine, pull out the wires, kick it and hit it and destroy it.

Instead, I blew my nose and sniffled and said politely to the attendants, 'I'm sorry.' As soon as I was dressed I repeated Monday's procedure. I read my vital statistics from that little white card in my cabinet.

Out in the Day Room I sat with Beverly. She had no memory

6

either. She complained to me with tears in her eyes of how she hated shock. I nodded with a few well-placed clucks and tsks-tsks. I felt as lousy as she did, but I won't let those nurses see it. If I don't control myself they'll write down things in my folder and Doctor Heineman will see it.

I'm sick, but I'm smart. Smart as I ever was. I know the right behaviour pattern here. Be good. I was good in school and good at camp and good at work, and I'll be good here. I'm lucky the nurses can't see behind my eyes, and that a shock machine is not a mind-reader. Just let me keep my mouth shut and a smile on my face.

Saturday, August 26

This morning Florence Adamski brought her accordion to the piano and accompanied Helen as she played some popular songs. Helen seems much better. When they took her out of solitary she was quiet and calm and completely rational. I wonder if she's smart like me.

She's so pretty. So tiny and small-boned. So full of fragile grace. She looks the way I've always wanted to look. Soft. Feminine. But it doesn't make any difference here. Josephine Hunter, that man-woman . . . Helen, whose face could fill a nineteenth-century cameo. And all the others in between.

Florence played beautifully this morning. I heard none of the fire raging from her private hell. She sang with us at the piano in a soft, husky voice, swaying easily, her stubby fingers caressing the accordion.

After lunch I lay down on my bed in one of the small wards off the hall. It's nice in this ward. I've been here since my first shock treatment. I hope they don't move me. My bed is next to the window. I like to watch the sunlight splatter through the bars and break into prisms of colour, and follow the dust motes dancing down the streams of light.

I was tired. I'm always tired. If not from shock, then from the constant tension that weights me down like the Old Man of the Sea. Suddenly, before I could stop it, I plunged into a kind of waking nightmare, something I haven't experienced since I was a child. Huge, billowing elephant-clouds were merging into a gigantic mass, growing larger and blacker as they moved in on me. A juggernaut of formless shapes rolling in from every corner of space, choking out light and air. A heavy, pressing pain, pushing and crushing, bringing Death unless I jump up and blink my eyes and keep blinking until the blackness disappears.

I rolled off the bed and stumbled to my feet, panting in fear and relief. I ran back to the Day Room, walked back and forth, struck up quick conversations with the women, forced words and laughter to my lips, all the while blinking away the shreds of clouds still lurking behind my eyes.

What the hell is the meaning in this formless wave of terror? No faces, no voices, no substance. I wish I could speak to a doctor about this. I have been here almost a month. Except for the two interviews with Doctor Manning, once when I was admitted and again when I cut my neck, no one has talked to me.

Sunday, August 27

Visiting day again. Felt much better seeing Jay. The two hours were like two minutes, a marathon of talking. I was telling him that I wanted to see Dr. Downey again when I got out, and my father interrupted with 'When, darling? When are you coming home?'

I answered him sharply.

'Just because I said I want to see the Doctor again doesn't mean I'm coming home, does it? Don't you think I'd tell you?'

He seemed to shrink into himself.

Why do I hurt him? Because his face and voice display all the feelings, all the anxiety, the despair, the hope, the disappointment, that I feel but cannot express? Because he loves me so much and shows it?

'I think it would be a very good idea', Jay said. 'I saw him at the hospital last week and he asked about you.'

'That's nice', I said, and thought with a rush of bitterness, *how considerate. How sweet. And he'll be so happy to take my money again when I come home, so ready with the words he trots out for his patients that come and go. Some go, like me, and never come back. Does he care? Does he know how I've suffered here? I hate him. I hate everyone who is well.* 'Will he help me? He didn't help me before.'

'That was before, sweetie. You're getting better. You'll be

calmer when you see him. You'll be more amenable to therapy.'

'I hope you're right.'

'I know I am. You'll get well. Just give it time. These things take time, sweetie.' He was smiling.

I wanted to pass my hands over his face, as the blind do, and feel his strength flow through my fingers.

'I feel angry towards him.'

'Who?'

'Dr. Downey. Because he didn't stop the breakdown. And other things.'

'So. Hostility towards your psychiatrist, huh? Very normal. Very normal.'

He stroked an imaginary beard under his chin in a mock gesture of sagacity. I laughed.

When I looked at my father he began to chuckle. I knew he didn't understand the joke. He laughed only because I did. And again I writhed with annoyance.

Don't puppy-dog me, Daddy. Don't be so anxious to please. Don't be so good to me. I'm not good. You make me feel like a little child when I want to be big and grown up. But I don't know how.

Why do I wait and wait for visiting days to see my father and husband and then waste precious moments talking to myself instead of to them?

'Jay, how do I find out what's wrong with me? Why I had a breakdown? Why I'm afraid of everything? Why——?'

'Therapy. Or analysis.'

'Can I be analysed?'

'Yes. If you want to.'

'It's expensive.'

'We could manage it.'

'Are you sure?'

'I'm sure. But let's wait a while. Until after you come home. We'll see how things go.'

'They won't go well, I know it. Jay, Dad, I'm scared stiff of that baby.'

'It'll subside. You just have to give it time.'

'That's right, darling.' My father leaned towards me and patted my hand.

'Time, time.'

'O.K. *O.K.*, *O.K.!*' I yelled at them. 'You'll see, I won't get better. I'll never get out of here.'

'Is that what you want?' Jay asked.

I slumped in the chair. 'I have no courage. No strength. I don't know what happened, and when you can't understand a thing how can you fight it?'

- 'Are you better now than before electro-shock?'

'Yes. But that's just for the depression, isn't it?'

'You're going to have therapy when you come home. Don't forget that. And . . . I know you don't like the word . . . but time will help.'

'Rome wasn't built in a day', my father said.

'Who the hell cares about Rome? What time is it?'

Jay looked at his watch. 'Ten to eleven.'

'It's almost over.'

'Yes. Do you want us to leave now?'

'Why do you say that?'

'You're annoyed with us.'

'No. I'm annoyed with myself. I just want to know what's wrong with me.'

'You will. Believe me, sweetie, you will. And you know something?'

'What?'

'You're getting better.'

Maybe he was right. Tonight, sitting in the Day Room and watching television, I suddenly wanted to get out of here. To be with Jay and the baby. To hold Gary. To look at him without fear. To sleep in my own bed. To open a door that is unlocked. To eat at my own kitchen table. I want to go home.

Monday, August 28

Someone else wanted to go home last night. Very badly.

She was a new patient, in our ward only two days. In the middle of the night she sat up in bed and screamed, 'Get me out of here! I want to get out of here', over and over, her voice rising to a keening wail.

Two nurses obliged. They pulled her out of bed and into the hall. She didn't come back this morning.

Disturbed patients make me so nervous. I'm afraid of the

torment inside them, as if they had a terrible disease that I might catch. This is stupid. And childish. But I can't help it.

I spent the rest of last night staring into the darkness. Jay is right. I *am* better than I was. The solid block of fear has broken into shreds and pieces of worry.

Will the baby accept me when I come home? How will I bathe him . . . my hands shake so badly. Suppose he crawls away when I am alone with him and eats poison and dies? How long can Mother stay with me? Dad is so lonely for her. Is Jay bluffing me? He really doesn't know whether I'll get well.

A hundred, a thousand, a million and one little fears. Like a school of fish they twist and wriggle and slither by in a never-ending stream.

Tuesday, August 29

They took us out this afternoon for almost two hours. I sat on the ground and felt the grass prickle my skin. I squinted at the yellow ball of sun in a sky washed clean of clouds. I pressed my hands against the ground and said, The world is good. I want to live.

'Hey, Judy! Look at my hair. Ain't it pretty? Don't the curls hang nice?'

Mary had plumped down next to me, spread-eagled her arms and legs and arched her neck, shaking a mass of curls in my face.

'Yes. Very pretty. Did you set it all by yourself?' She has slept with a dozen men and yet I talk to her as I would to a child.

'Yes. I did it this morning and I kept it up all this time so the curls would be tight.'

'You've got fresh make-up on, too.'

'Uh-huh.' She pulled up her skirt and wriggled her feet in the grass.

There was a yellow streak of powder under her chin. Her lipstick was thick and heavy and smelt like cherries.

I started to smile inside. Not at her. At me. For me. Suddenly I wanted to stand before a mirror and paint my face and fuss with my hair. It was the depression that made me turn away from mirrors. And pictures and beauty and living. Depression depresses. Relief relieves. And the ego springs back. Simple as that. But only when you're out of it.

A butterfly settled on the grass near Mary. We both watched it open and close its yellow wings.

'Judy, does the stuff come off them when you touch a butterfly?' Mary asked.

'Yes, I think so.'

'I'm going to get it. I want to see it die.'

'No, don't.' I slapped at her hand.

'I found a butterfly pin once. In a store. It was nice.'

'You found it or you took it?'

'I didn't take it.' She turned to me, her mouth in a pout. 'It fell off the counter and I picked it up. That's finding, isn't it?'

The butterfly opened its wings and flew upward, a tiny speck in the sunlight.

'When it comes back I'll get it and tear the wings off', Mary said.

'Well, I won't be here to see you.' I stood up.

'I don't care. I can do it by myself. I can do lots of things. I'm not afraid.'

When I sat down on the bench again, I turned to look at her, and thought, she's very sick. But she doesn't seem to know it. I wonder who is better off?

Wednesday, August 30

Slept very well last night with the earplugs Jay brought me.

For the first time in weeks I woke up free from tension. This is how it used to be when I was well, a thousand years ago. B.B. Before Baby. Before Breakdown.

They wake us up so damn early here. I nearly dozed sitting in the Day Room waiting for roll call.

More new admissions today. Strange voices answer to names I've never heard before. I don't like it. How do they expect me to keep track of everyone when they send in new patients each day? And they keep shifting my bed round. I never know where I'm going to sleep at night. The only thing I can be sure of is this knitting bag I carry on my arm. This diary is in there, too. I can't leave it in my cabinet any more. When I'm at the cafeteria one day they may clean out my cabinet to make room for a new patient.

Laura went home today. Yesterday, before she went to Staff, Bertha set her hair and helped her to dress. She hovered over her like a mother grooming her daughter for a prom. Bertha says it's important to look nice and neat when they take you to the doctors. Everyone dresses up for Staff. I suppose I will, too. I wonder when I'll go. Must have had ten shocks by now. They say if you're better after ten they take you off treatment. Otherwise they give you twenty. I don't know whether it's true. I scrounge information from other patients and student nurses.

We were waiting in the Day Room for Laura when she came back from Staff. I could see it in her eyes that she had passed. But she didn't seem excited. She smiled at Bertha and me. 'Well, what do you want to know?'

'How's the weather up there?' I teased.

'It's all right. I passed.'

'Oh, Laura! I'm so happy for you.' Bertha squeezed her and kissed her and patted her cheeks.

I hopped round her like a bug. 'Did they tell you you passed? What do they say? How do you know? Are there many doctors there? Do they ask many questions?'

'You do.' Laura laughed softly.

'I'm sorry', I said.

'It's all right. I know everyone is so anxious about Staff. I can't tell you much, Judith. Every patient is different.'

'But weren't you excited?'

'No. I've been there before. Now I had better find an attendant to pack my clothes. My mother is coming at three o'clock.'

'I know she'll be so happy, Laura', I said.

'Yes. She'll be happy. She loves me. God loves me, too. That's why I got well.'

'What will you do? Go back to teaching?'

'I don't know. I've been here five months. I've been quite sick. I want to rest up for a while.'

'Laura, write me every week, please.' Bertha took her arm. 'You promise?'

'I promise.'

'You won't forget?'

'No, I won't forget.' Then she called to me over her shoulder as they walked away. 'Judith, before I go, would you give me your home address?'

'Why?'

'I want to write to you, too. I want to keep in touch with all the friends I've made.'

When *I* go, I won't take one name, one address. She wants to remember . . . *I* want to forget.

Thursday, August 31

Sunday, Sunday, Sunday, can hardly wait for Sunday. I'm going home for one day. It's a start, a beginning. They're testing me. Trying me out.

Mrs. O'Neill told me the news this morning and stalked away before I could thank her. No, not really thank her, but ask questions. Who made the decision? Doctor Heineman? Will I go home every Sunday now? Does this mean I'm off shock? Will I soon go to Staff?

I have to keep hold. If I pester her and the others, they may cancel the pass.

Beverly saw me in the Day Room. I must have been smiling to myself.

'Good news?' she said.

'Yes. I'm going home Sunday.'

'For good?' Before I could answer she said, 'You're lucky. I always knew you were lucky. I have no luck. I never did.'

'Bev, it's just for the day. And I'm not so lucky. If I were, I wouldn't be here.'

'You won't stay much longer, Judy. First they let you go home Sundays. Then they give you a week-end pass. Then you go to Staff. Will you write to me, Judith?'

In spite of her eyes, I laughed. 'Beverly, please. Not so fast.'

'That's all right. I know. I'll be here when you go.' Her eyes brimmed with tears. 'I want to run away but I can't get out.'

'So do I.'

'Oh, no. Don't do that. It'll go bad for you. They won't give you the pass.'

'Don't worry. I won't be foolish.'

Foolish? Crazy. Real crazy. Maybe she's crazy to think of such an absurdity. Be cautious. Be careful. These words burn like torches in my head. They never go out. I won't let them.

Beverly looked so unhappy I was sorry I had told her about my Sunday.

'You'll go home soon, Bev. I know you will. We're both getting better.'

'I don't feel better. Much. And I hate shock treatment.'

'So do I. But don't you think it's helped?'

'I still hate it.'

'Let's find Bertha. We can play some cards.'

'I don't feel like playing cards.'

'Then we can sit and talk. Come on.' She got up and put her hand through mine. It was cold.

As we walked through the Day Room I thought, *Strange— ironic and strange. I am giving comfort and support when I can barely stand alone. The lame shall lead the blind.*

Friday, September 1

Something new and annoying. Incessant thoughts. Like a pulse. Like a rhythm. Home on Sunday . . . how will I do . . . must come through . . . how will I do? . . . Today is Friday . . . Friday fish . . . Saturday soup . . . Sunday chicken . . . Mother will cook chicken for me . . . with the carrots and celery swimming around in the golden fat . . . She'll stand and fix and stir and mix, her face wreathed in a cloud of steam as she bends over the pot, daring the soup to be watery or the chicken to be tough.

I can see her and the baby and Jay and my father. See them and hear them and feel them close, and I'm excited and scared. My pulse is up to 110. My palms are dripping. I'm bubbling and boiling like Mother's soup. I can't sit still. Ants in the pants and bugs in the brain.

Saturday, September 2

Now I have diarrhœa. I run to the bathroom every few hours. And it wakes me up at night. My knitting bag is stuffed with toilet paper. And I can't seem to stop that stream of rhythm words in my head. It's as though I were split in two; one part of me for communicating with the environment, the other for talking to myself. I hear a snatch of song on the television. Immediately my brain picks it up and repeats it endlessly, senselessly, just like a cracked gramophone record. A nurse calls out, 'Five minutes for cafeteria.' And I walk through the wards sing-songing inside, *Five and five for cafeteria . . . line up, girls, girls with curls . . . teria, leria, cafeteria . . .*

I feel like a coil spring wound too tight. I must be nervous. Terribly nervous. About tomorrow.

Sunday p.m., September 3

I don't have much time. They're going to put the light out in ten minutes and I must get everything down.

They let me wait for Jay this morning in the Day Room. I was wearing one of my own dresses. I didn't want to, but Millie made me put it on. She's the attendant in charge of patients' clothes.

'Judith, you ain't goin' home in a state dress, are you? You got nice dresses in your bin. I seen them. You're goin' to wear a nice fresh dress. Now you come back to the ward with me. I'll bring you a pretty one.'

She helped me into a cotton print.

'Beats me why you don't wear your own clothes.' She walked away, shaking her head.

I couldn't tell her I'm afraid of my clothes. You have to keep ahead of your things. Must wear less and dirty less and wash and iron less to save time. Never enough time. It's better not to use them. Let them collect in piles.

Waiting in the Day Room with my bulging knitting bag, I felt like an immigrant, expecting a relative to take me to a strange home. That was the trouble. I couldn't remember the layout of the apartment. And I hate the unknown. Maybe that's why I detest shock so much.

As he stepped off the lift I felt that nervous shudder in my stomach. It's always been like that for the first instant of our meetings.

'Hello, Jay.'

'Hello, sweetie. Are you all ready?'

'Wait a minute. I——'

'What?'

'Don't you want to talk?' I stalled.

'We can talk in the car. We'll save time that way.'

He's rushing me. Why doesn't he give me a chance for a little small talk . . . ease me into a thing like this?

'Are you glad I'm going home today?'

'Of course I'm glad.' He smiled and squeezed my hand. His was dry and warm. Mine dripped with clammy sweat. 'I told you last time you were getting better.'

'How did you find out about the pass?'

'They sent me a letter.'

'Who signed it?'

'The director of the hospital.'

'How does he know I'm better?'

'The doctors and nurses report to him. It's routine.'

'Doctor Heineman, do you think? Do you know him?'

'No. I haven't met him yet.' He touched my arm. 'Judy, we can talk about this in the car.'

'Don't be angry with me. I'm afraid.'

'I'm not angry. And I'm sorry—I didn't mean to rush you. Do you want to sit here a few minutes?'

'No. I'm O.K. Let's go.' I slipped my arm into his. 'I'm bringing my knitting bag, all right? I don't trust them here.'

I felt his arm stiffen. 'What do you mean, you don't trust them?'

'I have important things in here . . . cigarettes. Papers. Things like that. I have no place to leave them.'

'Oh.' He sounded relieved.

'And I've got three packets of toilet paper. I go to the bathroom so much.'

'Don't you think we have it at home?' He laughed.

'Yes. But the nursing office will be locked when I get back.'

He doesn't know. No one knows. How I think ahead and prepare myself for every eventuality. Everything but a breakdown. That wasn't in the plan.

When the lift stopped at the first floor I recognized the low-ceilinged reception room with the big table in the centre. I had said good-bye to him here so long ago. Now the room was crowded with visitors. Jay showed his pass to a nurse at the door and we walked through. All these weeks I had itched to see the outside. Now I couldn't lift my eyes. I stared at the gravel crunching under our feet.

'Here's the car, sweetie.'

'Is it still running O.K.?'

'Fine.' He opened the door for me. 'Happy?'

'Yes. I think so. But I'm nervous.'

'Don't worry about it. It's always like that the first time home.'

How do you know, my husband? My stranger husband. I split from you just as I did from everything else. And I'm still closer to the now than to the before.

He turned the ignition key and let the engine idle. 'Do you want to play the radio?'

'No.'

No music, please. Enough rhythm in my head as it is.

The car swung out between two stone pillars and then on to a main road. Look back, I told myself. Now's the time. You can see all the buildings and grounds. Instead, I studied the rubber floor mat and balled my hands into fists.

'How's everything at the hospital?'

'Pretty good. I'm busy, though. I'm on duty every second night. I don't get much sleep. Internship is rough.'

'Are you angry at me?'

'For what?'

'Getting sick now.'

'Don't talk like that. You didn't do it on purpose. It just happened. One thing, though. We'll never move right after we have a baby.'

'What makes you think I'll have another baby?'

Is he trying to torture me?

'Nice highway, isn't it?'

'Do you mind all this driving in one day?'

'No. It's not bad. It's a straight road all the way.'

Why couldn't you have said something else? Something sweet. Like, 'I'd drive twice as far to see you, darling.' Or, 'I'm bringing you home, sweetie. That's what counts.' Why don't you say nice things to me, to make me feel I'm not a bother and a trouble? My steady, sober, take-everything-in-stride husband. You adjust to everything, don't you? Even my breakdown. The wife is sick so he puts her in a hospital and carries on. He doesn't go to pieces. Why? WHY is he strong?

The road stretched ahead, cutting a swath through the green countryside. I remembered the pleasure I used to take in the grass and the sun and the sky. Today I couldn't bear to look at it. I rocked back and forth in the seat mumbling wordlessly.

Take me back . . . take me back . . . still rejecting . . . still hiding . . . still afraid . . . not ready to go home . . . hot in here . . . need some air . . . choking.

'Your mother'll have a good meal for us. She was shopping yesterday. She bought a lot of food.'

'How did she get out?'

'Your father doesn't work on Saturdays in the summer. Remember? He comes down Friday nights. Sweetie, are you worried about shopping and cooking and managing things with the baby?'

'Yes. I've been thinking about it all week.'

'When you're home for good you won't do everything at once. Your mother will stay as long as you need her. You'll work into things gradually.'

'Why am I different from other women? Why did I fall apart?'

'I don't know. Yet.'

'It wasn't a hormone disturbance, was it? That's what you said when I went to the hospital in Philadelphia.'

'I was trying to calm you. Are you sure you don't want the radio?'

'No. Jay, you'd better stop the car. I'm afraid. Of seeing the baby. I'm scared stiff.'

He eased the car on to the shoulder of the road. 'Darling, I don't think you really want to go back to the hospital. Try it. It's just for one day. See how it goes. O.K.?'

'All right. Start the car.'

'Maybe you'd like a soda or some ice-cream? We could stop off——'

'No. Go fast. Let's get there. Then I'll know.'

'Sweetie, I understand how you feel.'

Doyoudoyoudoyou.

My thoughts spun with the wheels. Happiness is mutual. Pain

is a private thing. . . . We talked very little for the rest of the trip. I sat hunched in the seat and didn't look up until he said, 'We're almost there. How do you feel?'

'All right.'

Fine. Marvellous. Great. Pulse must be up to 120.

He stopped the car in front of a row of homes. I clutched the knitting bag as he helped me out of the car.

'Which house?'

'This one. Ready?'

'Yes.'

We went up some steps to a porch. He had his hand on the door when it opened. My parents were standing in the hallway. My mother was wiping her hands on a dish towel, her eyes clouded with tears; Father was behind her.

'Hello, Mother. Daddy. Everything all right?'

She kissed me. 'So why shouldn't it be? You're home.' Her voice was shaky. And her face felt saggy and soft.

'Welcome home, darling', my father said. 'You all right?'

'Fine.' I took a few steps into the living-room. Then I turned to them. 'You know, I don't remember——'

And then I heard Jay whispering to them '. . . alone . . . nervous . . . don't push . . . questions . . .'

I walked through the living-room and the kitchen and then through another room. There was a crib and nappies piled on chairs, and a bathinette.

'Where is he?'

'In the bedroom', my father said. 'He just fell asleep. Oy, oy, oy!' He slapped his hand to his face and shook his head. 'What a baby you have!'

The bassinet was by the back door. I leaned over and looked down at a sleeping infant in a cotton shirt and checked plastic pants. The fists were tightly curled and the legs splayed out like those of a little frog.

Now, isn't that sweet? Such a precious little boy, It IS a boy, isn't it? Looks just like the father. I'm so happy for you. What? Oh, no, it isn't mine. It belongs to you two, standing there. Yes, you are a little old. You look more like grandparents than parents. But you'll take good care of him, won't you? You see, the real mother is afraid of him and doesn't want him. She tried to kill herself when he was born. She's sick.

*Yes, it's a shame. Well, I'll be going now. Maybe I'll drop in again. . . .
Good-bye.*

I said, 'I can't believe he's here. I'm going to the bathroom a
minute. I'll be right out.'

I closed the door.

*This room I remember. And that medicine chest. The box of sleeping
pills. Wonder if it's still there, or has Jay thrown them away? Never
mind. I don't want them now. I'm better. There's only one thing wrong.
I have no identification with that baby. They tell me it's mine and I
know it's mine. Physically. That's all. They're talking about me out
there. Jay must be briefing them on what to say and what not to say.
Humour her. Don't ask questions. Don't rave about the baby. . . . Be
patient with the patient. It's her first time home.*

As I opened the door I heard the baby cry. It frightened me,
but not as much as I imagined it would. My mother came
running.

'He's up, Daddy. He's up', she called to my father.

I hung back, watching Mother pick up my baby and cuddle
him. I thought, *how beautiful he is. Where do I come off to have such
a beautiful baby?*

'Do you want to hold him?' Jay was behind me, his hand on
my shoulder.

'Yes. I think so.'

'Frieda, let her hold him.'

'Whatever you say. I would have waited. I mean, I wouldn't
have come to him, but, Jay, you said not to push, I mean——'

'That's all right, Mother. I know what you mean.'

*She tries so hard to do the right thing. She always was that way.
So responsibility-ridden. And so am I.*

She gave me my baby. Warm. Tiny. So very tiny. Dark
brown eyes. Almost black. I thought he might cry out, but he
lay quietly in my arms. I shifted him carefully until his head
nestled in the crook of my elbow.

A flood of tears rushed to my eyes. I turned my face so they
couldn't see and wouldn't hear.

*My son. Forgive me. Forgive my fear, my hate, my rejection of you.
You are so beautiful and I am sick.*

I laid him down gently and fumbled for a handkerchief to
blow my nose.

'Mother, did you bathe him this morning?'

'No. Not yet. Do you want to?' She shot a glance at Jay. He nodded to her.

'Yes, I want to.'

He started to whimper. I lifted him to my shoulder and patted his back.

'You were good at that, remember?' my mother said. 'You knew how to handle him and put his nappy on. You even cut his nails. I still can't do that. I'm afraid.'

'Let's get the bath ready.' No point in telling them that shock had swept my mind clean, had neatly obliterated the recent past. As I walked with him through the house I saw drying wash and nappies, cans of formula, vitamin drops, bottles . . . all the infant paraphernalia that had risen like spectres to overwhelm and terrorize.

I closed my eyes and chewed my lips. No. Not today. I won't let the bogeys out. Later, perhaps. Back in the hospital. But not now. I sat down in the kitchen while my mother prepared his bath and held Gary close to me, my body rocking back and forth and my throat making little cooing sounds. Ah . . . aah . . . ba-bee, sweet, lit-tle ba-bee . . .

The night nurse is checking the ward. She'll put out the light in a few minutes. I'm writing so fast I doubt if I'll be able to read this. But that's all right. I won't forget this day.

I carried my son round the house. I bathed him, fed him, changed him. Mother was always there, handing me things and helping me. I couldn't tell her, but she made me nervous. She meant well. She always does. But there's a tension in her. It charges the air like electricity and falls on me in a shower of sparks.

Why do I criticize? My mother is keeping my home together. If it weren't for her, Jay would have to board the baby in a foster home.

Coming back in the car, my three horsemen began to ride again. I call them Anticipation, Apprehension, and Anxiety. All day I had held them in check. Now I was tired, I thought, did I really see my son? Did I wash the dishes in my own house? Was I happy for those eight hours? Or did I perform a role in

7

a short play, doing what was expected of me, without true feeling or volition? Do I really want to go back there again?

'I'm nervous, Jay. Just like this morning. Why?'

'I don't know, sweetie. Maybe it's the strain of the day. It was your first time home, you know. I think you did very well.' He patted my leg. I moved closer to him.

'I need you.'

'I'm here. I always will be. I love you. Don't forget it.'

'Thank you.'

'For what?'

'For loving me.'

'We're almost there.' He swung the car on to the gravel road and parked in front of the building.

'Is there time to sit here a few minutes before we go in?'

'I don't think so. It's ten minutes to eight.'

As we walked to the door I saw a young girl coming up the path with her parents. A nurse called out to us, 'Have a nice time, girls?'

'Fine! Fine', we answered in unison, and looked at each other in embarrassment. She kissed her parents hurriedly and went to the lift. I took Jay's hand in mine and squeezed it. 'Write me.' My voice was choked and husky.

'Of course I will.' He spoke low. 'I'll come for you next Sunday.'

'Will I have another pass?'

'I don't see why not.' Then his lips framed the words, 'I love you', and he winked at me as he pulled his hand away.

When I stepped off the lift the Day Room was crowded. They were all watching television. Food packages were open on the tables and I saw the Sunday newspapers scattered around. The smell of candy and over-ripe fruit was strong.

A feeling of comfort enveloped me, a feeling of safety in returning to the known and the familiar. This is *my* hospital, I thought. Until today it had been The Hospital, This Place. Now the great fear had lost its giant grip. I think I was even a little glad to be back. I had had enough of home for one day. I had tried so hard. Now I was tired.

Darkness crept through the wards, capping the summer twilight. I walked to the washroom, took out my cigarettes,

and looked for my friends. I wanted to see them before I went
to bed.

Monday, September 4

*No more pencils, no more books . . . no more teachers' dirty looks . . .
feeling great . . . feeling swell . . . shock machine can go to hell . . .*

I was sitting in the Day Room, flipping the pages of a film
magazine. On the cover was written in a childish hand, 'This
Belongs Too Mary'.

'I'll be sitting here and reading, I thought, when they wheel
the shock machine down this aisle . . . so close I could touch it
. . . but I won't. I'll have my eyes on this book and I won't look
up . . . It's not for me. I'm finished. I'm through. I've had mine.
Thank God it's over.

*See? It's good to keep a record. Last night I checked back in my
diary and counted up my shock treatments. I had ten. Now I'm off
treatment—that's what they all told me. If you improve with ten they
put you on observation to see how you behave . . . oh, they won't have
any trouble with me . . . the very very model of a model little patient . . .
so happy I could scream or cry or dance . . . now look what Mary did to
this film star . . . put a moustache on her . . . silly . . . funny . . . everything's funny . . .*

'Judith. I thought you were undressed. Hurry up. This is
Monday, you know.' Mrs. O'Neill startled me. I stood up,
knocking the magazine to the floor.

'Oh, no. There's a mistake, Mrs. O'Neill. I've had ten treatments. I keep a list. I have it right here.' I fumbled in my
knitting bag for my diary, tossing out wads of tissues and toilet
paper. 'You've made a mistake——'

'There's no mistake. You only had nine. We have lists, too.'

'Ten!'

She took my arm firmly and led me to the big ward. 'Now
don't argue with me. You're down for shock today. When
Doctor Heineman comes, you can talk to him.'

'It'll be too late. He'll give it to me anyway. Let me wait here
for him, please.'

'We follow orders here', she said. 'Get undressed and get into
bed.'

She kicked the door closed behind her.

'Here's the last one', she called to the student nurses. 'Help her undress.' She walked away.

I stood there shaking my head and wiping away tears.

'What's the matter, Judith?' One of the students put her arm round my waist.

'I'm not supposed to have shock today. I've had ten. I have it all marked down. She's making a big mistake.'

'Now why don't you take it today? It will probably be your last one.'

'If I get in bed, and Doctor Heineman says I don't have to take shock, could I get dressed again?'

'Sure.'

'All right.' I walked with her to the bathroom, shame burning my cheeks.

'What happened?' Beverly had the bed next to mine. 'I saw you crying.'

'Nothing. I'm all right now.'

I forced myself to lie quietly while they moved the shock machine from bed to bed. When he came to me I sat up.

'Doctor Heineman, do I have to take shock today?'

'Of course.'

'But I've had ten. Isn't that when you stop?'

'Sometimes yes. Sometimes no. Lie down, please.'

'Will this be the last one? Will it?'

'From now on once a week. On Monday.'

'But I thought——'

'I am sorry, Judith. Now you lie down.'

No fear this time. No hate. Just blind tears and hopeless resignation.

And now I'm ashamed. I've acted like a child. I've broken control and made my first false step. Their weapon is authority. I have nothing to match that. I must be docile, bending, meek, and willing.

Tuesday, September 5

Every morning now I brush my hair and put on make-up. There are only two mirrors in the entire ward. I use the one in the small utility room where I slept the first few nights I was here.

I like to see Anna come in and watch her loosen the plaits of her long hair. She holds them in front of her and brushes with careful strokes and then coils them up again high on her head. This morning I talked with her after most of the other patients had left.

'I'm feeling better these days, Anna.'

'It is easy to see that. I told you you would get better. Remember? You were not much for believing me—you were crying all the time.'

I must have looked embarrassed. She took my hands in hers. 'You are a nice girl. You will go home soon.'

'How about you?'

She shrugged. 'We will see. So far there is no place for me. The State is making arrangements. When I do not know. My children write to me. I want to be with them. With money I could make a home again. But I have no money. If I did not know that God has a reason for everything that happens I would feel no good inside.' She thumped her chest with her fist.

Then she patted her hair, pushing down a final hairpin. 'So! Finished.'

As she walked past me she said, 'You are a lucky girl, Judith. Remember: in everything bad there is good. I will see you again.'

This afternoon I was sitting by the outside door waiting for Miss Willems. She came along jingling her keys and sang out, 'Who wants nice fresh air?'

'I'll buy that', I quipped. 'How much?'

'Honey, today you go to O.T.'

'O.T.?'

'Occupational therapy. Wait by the other door. Miss McAllister'll be here soon. She'll take you over.'

'Will I be the only one?'

'No. There are some more going from A Ward. And you'll meet other girls there. You'll like it.' She put a cool hand on my arm.

My hands began to shake again. I thought, another test. I will have to produce something creative, and they will judge me. I can't work with these shaking hands. They're useless.

Helen came over and sat next to me, and then Thelma came.
I call her the jigsaw girl. I don't like her. She's not friendly. She
never talks unless you talk first and then she uses sentences
without cues for further conversation.

I turned to Helen. 'Are you going to O.T.?'

'Yes. Can you make things? I'm afraid. I'm not good with my
hands.' She folded her tiny hands and plumped them up and
down in her lap. 'I wish I didn't have to go.'

*Helen, Helen, I love you. You're frightened, too, and that makes
me feel strong so I can bluff the fear for both of us.*

'Oh, I think it might be fun. Look, we'll both start on the
same thing so we can help each other. O.K.?'

Her china-blue eyes flashed a thank-you smile.

A key turned in the door, and a tall, thin woman came in.
She carried a large clipboard and I was reminded of the camp
counsellors. I expected to see a whistle hanging from her neck.
Miss Willems called out, 'That's Miss McAllister, girls.'

'Hello, girls.'

'Hello, Miss McAllister.' We sounded like children greeting a
new teacher.

'This is Thelma and Helen and Judith.'

'Are these the only ones today?' Miss McAllister said.

'That's it.'

'All right. I'll bring them back at four. Shall we go,
girls?'

We followed her down the steps. We were at the rear of the
building. We crunched on gravel past garbage cans and garden
tools. I smelt food and knew that the kitchen must be near-by.
And I saw a tall smokestack jutting from a building.

'Miss McAllister, is that the laundry?' I asked.

'Yes, Helen.'

'I'm Judith.'

'Oh.' She laughed. 'I never can get the names right off. And
when I get to know you girls you go home. You've never been
along this way, have you?'

'No', I answered. Helen and Thelma were quiet. I was doing
all the talking. (*I talk a lot lately. I'm full of pep. Nervous pep. As
though I'd had a shot of adrenalin. I tingle and bubble inside.*) 'This
hospital is very big, isn't it?' I continued.

'Oh, dear me, yes. It took me quite a while to find my way round.' She walked briskly with long strides. We found it hard to keep up with her. 'Here we are, girls.'

It was dark and rather cool inside the building, and the place smelt of paint and lacquer and freshly shaved wood. Picture frames were hanging on the walls and hammered copper plaques were propped up on long wooden tables. Brushes were drying in paint-spattered tin cans. Tiny scraps of leather and wool littered the floor.

A few women were working with leather punches at a long table. I was about to go over to them when Miss McAllister said, 'Try the loom for today.'

'What?'

'The loom. Weaving. Sit down over there. I'll be right with you. Helen and Thelma, come this way.'

Helen looked frightened. 'Can't we all do the same thing?'

'I think it's more interesting if you each try something different, don't you, Helen?'

She didn't answer. I knew how scared she was. And I was too. The weaving loom looked monstrous. I eased myself up on a seat and stared at the heavy frame. I thought, *if she thinks I'm going to make anything on this she's crazy. I don't know a warp from a woof from a hole in the wall. I'm nervous. Do they have a bathroom here? Maybe she'll forget about me. Wonder what Helen's doing? Can't see her from here . . . Thelma's probably on a jigsaw puzzle . . . seat is so high . . . can't reach the treadle . . . or is it a spindle? no, spindle holds spool of wool . . . hell! Of all the damn things, she had to assign me to weaving . . . why couldn't I fingerpaint or bang on copper?*

When she came over to me I said, 'Miss McAllister, I don't know the first thing about a loom.'

'Then it should be fun.'

'Do we get grades for the things we do?'

'Oh, dear me, no. Now watch me. We're making a rug. Most of it is finished. See? There it is in the roller.'

'Who made all that?'

'Other patients. If you finish it you can buy it. (*That's what she thinks. When I leave I want no mementoes.*) Now here we go', she sang out, cheerily. 'You carry the spindle . . . push down on the treadle . . . this is the woof . . . pack it back tight with the paddle

. . . now come back the other way. See? Now take your time . . .
I'll check you in a little while.'

I worked. Pushing, pulling, threading. My hands shook badly
and my head ached with the effort to remember her instructions. In the hour we were there I called her over at least five
times and had to repeat three rows. I had woven six tight and
lumpy rows.

And yet, when I was back in the ward, I felt a thrill of pride
thinking of my work. I had used my mind and hands for something other than worry. And I was anxious to return to O.T.

Wednesday, September 6

Am sleeping quite well lately. Of course the moment I awake
I run to the bathroom for my daily diarrhœa. But that's all
right. I know it's from tension and I can tolerate it. Beverly
complains of constant headaches. Gloria still has those pains in
her stomach. Many of the other women lie on their beds most
of the day. They say they're tired.

Yet the only one who really looks bad is Connie. She has a
terrible skin condition. I think it's psoriasis. Yet they give her
nothing to relieve the itching. She scratches those red patches
on her face and arms until they ooze blood. I feel so sorry for
her. Not just for her rash, but because she is so sick. I know
she'll be here a long time.

Other than going to the cafeteria, she spends all her time in
the bathroom, sitting on the toilet, curling long strands of hair
over her fingers. She's very dirty. I've never seen her wash.
Her state dress is ripped and it has no buttons or belt. She walks
around in house slippers. Her nails are crusted with grime, and
the sight and the sound of them scratching, scratching makes
me nauseous. She rocks back and forth on that toilet crooning
in a monotone, 'when I go home . . . when I go home . . .
they'll come for me soon . . . yes, they will . . . soon oh soon
. . . when I go home . . .'

She hears us talking and words like Staff and Parole and
Week-end Pass excite her to a frenzy of mumbling . . . Yes
oh yes, I'm going to Staff . . . then I'll go home . . . they'll
come for me . . . you'll see . . .'

We don't see. We shut her out from our conversations and

turn our backs when we light up cigarettes. She's always scrounging cigarettes, begging with her eyes. At first I would give her one every time I came into the bathroom. Then Esther took me aside and said, 'Look, kid, she'll drain you dry. She has smokes. I don't know where she gets them, but she has them. I saw a full packet in her pocket yesterday. She don't give us and she's always grubbing. Hand her your butt once in a while. That's all.'

'But it's so hard to say no. She's——'

'Look. Here you have to do what's good for *you*, understand?' Esther jabbed my chest with her finger. 'They don't think we got heads around here. Why should we have hearts?' She pointed to Connie. 'She's looney, that one. She was here before I came and I've been here six months. She's going home like that bucket over there is going home. I wish to hell she'd stop that scratching.'

This morning a woman came through the Day Room wheeling a cart filled with books. I went over to her.

'Would you like to read a book? We have some recent best-sellers here.'

'I don't know. (*Could I stop the marathon, the sing-song merry-go-round in my head and concentrate?*) How long can I keep a book?'

'Two weeks. You can renew, of course. I come by here every week.'

I ran my hands over the covers, fingering and fondling and feeling hunger. The cart looked liked the kind they used in libraries. But here I had no time to thumb through pages and juggle one title against the other.

Pick one, any one—she won't stand there all day and wait for you. She'll get angry and go away.

My hand closed over a thin volume. Without reading the title, I said, 'I'll take this one. Do I sign a card?'

'No, that's all right.'

I was disappointed. I wanted a library card. I wanted to see my name on something other than a treatment chart or an electro-shock tag.

Thursday, September 7

I lay in bed this morning and I imagined I was home. The

house was empty and still. Then I heard the baby cry. I lifted him from the bassinet and cradled him in my arms, my body throbbing with the thrill of possession. My hands explored the folds of the blanket, looking for him. When I opened my eyes I·knew I hadn't been dreaming. It was a deliberate make-believe, a wish-fantasy I had created.

I want to think that this is a good sign. But I'm afraid to generalize about my emotions. I swing from high to low in a matter of minutes. I teeter on a mental see-saw, rising to heights of breezy confidence only to fall back into fear and apprehension.

I was making my bed after breakfast when I sensed someone standing next to me. It was Doctor Connor. He was wearing that same brown suit and his hands were shoved deep in the pockets. His yellow hair and the freckles on his face gave him the appearance of a schoolboy.

'Hullo, Judith. Can I talk to you for a minute?'

What did I do? What's wrong? Why did he come like this?

He sat on the bed, crossed one leg over the other knee, and held on to his ankle. I stared at the freckles on the back of his hand.

'We want to speak to your husband.'

'Why? I mean, what about?'

Going home? Maybe? But he's not smiling.

'You seem to have developed an excitable type of personality. We want to find out from him if that's normal for you.'

'Excitable? What do you mean, Doctor Connor?' My mouth went dry and hot.

'You're behaving very differently now. You're very bright. Too bright. You're always joking and laughing and you're full of energy. That's quite a change from a few weeks ago, don't you think? We just wonder if this is a phase of your normal personality.'

'Oh, yes. Yes, Doctor Connor. This is how I am. Really. (*I knew it. They watch you here. Watch you all the time. How you look, how you talk . . . if you never laugh . . . or laugh too much. Did I make a mistake? I thought I've been showing them how much I've improved.*) You have me all wrong. This *is* my normal way. The shock treatments worked. They were very good for me. Oh, yes. Very good. They brought me round. I feel so much better now. I'm out of the depression. I make jokes because I feel so good. I'm not excitable. I'm not a manic-depressive. That's what you meant, wasn't it?'

Fool. Why did you use that word? You've put a bug in his ear.

He stood up. 'Well, we just want to make sure, that's all. We want to hear what your husband has to say about you. Now don't worry about it. By the way, you know we're continuing shock for you once a week?'

'Yes. Doctor Heineman told me. (*Did they tell him what a fuss I made?*) But don't you have to be off shock to go home?'

'No. Sometimes we give shock on a Monday and the patient goes to Staff on Friday. There's no set rule.'

I tried frantically to think of more questions. I talk to a doctor so seldom, and now I couldn't think straight.

'You'd better finish your bed now.' He walked to the door. 'I'll see you again.'

'When will you see my husband?'

'Some time next week. He's interning now, isn't he?'

'Yes. It's hard for him to get here.'

'We'll make some arrangements. Good-bye, Judith.'

I stood by the bed, fingering the spread, and thought, this is bad. Very bad. A turn I hadn't planned on. They think I'm manic. Have to get word to Jay. Warn him. Tell him to be careful and say the right things. Last Sunday was the first time we've been together in months. He may be confused about me . . . may hesitate . . . sound indecisive. A letter. Have to write him a letter. . . . But they censor the mail . . . they read every word . . . maybe a phone call . . . do they ever let patients call home? . . . oh, God, to do something.

I walked out to the Day Room. Bertha was sitting there playing solitaire. I mumbled to her perfunctorily and sat down. The worry must have shown on my face.

'What's the matter, Judy?'

Don't say anything. She may tell someone else. She's chummy with the student nurse. Oh, what the hell!

'Doctor Connor told me they're going to speak to Jay next week. They think I'm acting funny. Too peppy. Different from when I came. They want to know what's my normal behaviour.'

'Are we supposed to be here if we're normal?' She winked and continued to turn up the cards.

'Don't tease me, Bertha. Please. I have to tell Jay about this. Tell him what to say. And he won't be here this Sunday.'

'You can't write a letter. They read them.'

'I know. I know.'

'Not the regular way.'

'What do you mean?'

'Talk low. I have an idea.' She shifted her eyes and then hunched over the table, her plump breasts swelling from the neck of her dress.

'What idea?'

'I said keep your voice down. Now pick up these cards and shuffle them and listen while I talk.'

'I can't. I'm too nervous. I'll spill them all over.'

'Then just fiddle with them. I know somebody. I can get a letter out for you. A private letter. It won't go through the nursing office. It'll go direct. You can write anything you want. How's that?' She leaned back and patted her head, feeling for loose hair grips under her kerchief.

I looked at her and thought, she's lying. Making this whole thing up. Playing with me.

'Are you sure, Bertha? You really do know someone here who——'

Her fat face sagged. 'Would I lie to you, Judy? You're my friend. Now write the letter.'

'Let me do it back in the ward. I can think better there.'

'O.K. But don't let them see you. I'll wait in the small toilet next to the nursing office.'

Friday, September 8

It seems as though the entire staff knows Jay is coming to talk to the doctors. When I checked in with the technician after breakfast this morning, she closed her roll book and walked with me up the ward aisle.

'How are you doing?' she asked.

'Fine, Miss Quinn.'

'You made a fuss about shock on Monday, didn't you? Why?'

'I . . . I thought I'd had ten shocks . . . that I'd graduated, you know?' I giggled nervously.

'There's no set rule here. We go by the patient's progress. Personally—and this is my own opinion, mind you—I think your behaviour made Doctor Heineman wonder about you. Whether you're ready to go off shock. Well, we'll see what happens when they talk to your husband.' She patted my shoulder. 'Now don't worry about it. Go help the girls straighten up the Day Room.'

Don't worry don't worry. They scare me and tell me not to worry. Almost a hundred patients here and they watch me like hawks. Can't I get upset a little? Or laugh a lot? I'm a patient here. I'm sick. What do they want from me?

Saturday a.m., September 9

Very little time to write. Jay will be here in a few minutes. Am going home for the week-end.

Can't believe it and can't understand it. Thought my recent behaviour cancelled out visits home. A full week-end pass was inconceivable. Yet five minutes ago Mrs. O'Neill tells me 'your husband is coming for you this morning. You're going home for the week-end. Stay in the Day Room where we can find you.'

Can't figure them out and am not going to try. All that worry. That frantic conspiracy with Bertha. Completely unnecessary. But who would have dreamed this could happen? Feel like a chess pawn. Have to find Bertha and tell her the news. Then get the attendant. This state dress is soiled. I want a clean one. One of my own. I want to look pretty for Jay.

Sunday, September 10

Spent most of the past 36 hours telling them 'I can't believe I'm home . . . it's so hard to realize I slept in my own bed . . . Jay . . . Mother . . . Dad . . . it seems so strange to be home . . .'

Yet I did fairly well. I took care of Gary. Washed a few of his clothes. Even helped make the salad for Saturday supper. But my eyes never rested and the questions never stopped. I think all my mutterings of 'Isn't it strange?' were bubbles of fear breaking to the surface and all those 'Can't-believes' meant 'Won't believe'. This worries me. Am I really ready for release?

They wouldn't send me home each week if they had no plans for me.

Am I strong enough? Will I have a relapse a few days after I'm released? What are the long-range effects of a shock cure?

As I walked off the lift tonight I saw a woman who looked familiar. I recognized her face and her red hair. But she wasn't in the ward when I left on Saturday. I found Bertha up near the television set.

'Well, hello! Did you have a good time?'

'Fine. Fine. Say, I——'

'Did you talk to Jay about it?' she whispered. 'You know what I mean.'

'Yes. It'll be all right. He knows what to say. Bertha, do you know——'

'How's the baby?'

'Fine. Very cute. I took care of him a little. He's three months old already.'

'I like them young, don't you? They're so helpless. They need love. Lots of love.'

'Oh, you're right. Definitely. Listen, who's that red-haired woman standing there near the lift? She's talking to a nurse.'

'That's Roslyn.'

'Wasn't she here before?'

'Yes. They sent her home a few days after you came.'

'Then why——?'

'She came back Saturday. That's all I know.'

'She got sick again, didn't she?'

'I guess so. Why are you so interested?'

'Nothing. It's just a shame. I hate to see anyone come back.'

Will it happen to me? Will it?

'Look, doll. This place is like Grand Central station. People come and go. You can't worry about all of them.'

'When I get out, I hope I don't come back.'

'Well, so do I! Tell me more about your baby. Who does he look like, you or Jay?'

'Me, I think. How about yours?'

'Oh, I don't know. She doesn't look like either of us. Look, we're missing a good show. Let's watch TV.'

Monday, September 11

The news spread like fire. I heard it first in the washroom after breakfast. Esther walked in and clapped the woman nearest her on the shoulder.

'Girls, we been reprieved. We been commuted. No shock today.'

I rushed to her. 'Are you sure? Who told you? Nobody gets it? Are you sure?'

'Sure I'm sure.'

'But who told you?' I pressed her.

'A nurse. Who do you think, my weejee board?'

'Which nurse?'

'How the hell do I know? One of them hanging around the office.'

I rushed out to the office.

'Mrs. O'Neill, can I ask you a question? I heard. I mean, the girls said . . . there's no shock today?'

'That's right. No treatment today. Unless you want it.' The lines of her face loosened in a little smile.

'Oh, no. I mean——'

'You're glad, aren't you?'

I eased myself out, gesturing vaguely. 'It doesn't make much difference, really.' The lie came so easily. 'I just wanted to be sure, that's all. Thank you, Mrs. O'Neill.'

I went into the small washroom to smoke and watched a patient scrub out the sinks. She worked hard, rubbing scouring powder into the dark discolorations.

'Why knock yourself out like that?' I asked her. 'It's a holiday.' I felt flippant.

'You never do any work around here any time,' she snapped back, 'holiday or no holiday.' She wrung out the rag, hung it over the side of the sink, and stamped out.

Why the hell should it bother her? I'm not the only one. Scrubbing sinks and mopping floors won't get me out of here any faster. They're all suckers the way they break their backs every morning.

Twenty minutes later I was washing the walls of the Day Room, sweat pouring down my back and forehead and fogging my glasses.

Miss Spence is back from a six-weeks' leave. Adelaide Spence.

Head attendant. Veteran employee. Major-domo. Martinet. And a bitch.

I heard her before I saw her. A loud, metallic voice rang in the corridor.

'Where are my attendants? Where are they? I want everyone on day shift in the office in five minutes. This ward is filthy. Filthy!'

I poked my head out of the bathroom and saw a tall woman standing with her legs spread apart and her hands planted on her hips. She was talking to two attendants who looked awed and frightened. She turned and I saw a long, angular face with the skin stretched taut over bony cheekbones and across a high forehead. She wore no make-up and her faded blonde hair was tightly curled under a net. The skirt of her starched uniform stood out from her body like a crinoline, and her white shoes were spotless. She looked antiseptic.

Just as I moved back into the bathroom a student nurse passed by. I motioned her in. 'Who is that . . . that woman?' I pointed outside.

She laughed. '*That* is Miss Adelaide Spence.'

'Which makes me . . .?' I still felt chipper.

'A very unfortunate girl, Judy. You and all the others. From now on, no smoking in the toilets, no loafing during clean-up, no lying on the beds.'

'But she's just an attendant, isn't she?'

'Head attendant. Even the nurses don't cross her', she whispered.

'Brr.' I shivered in mock terror.

'It's not funny, girl. I'm glad I'll be off A Ward in a week. Now I've got to run. I've got a pan of needles to sterilize. Doctor Manning is coming back tomorrow and we start insulin shock again. 'Bye.'

I tip-toed out of the bathroom. Miss Spence was standing in the doorway of the office, checking off items from a clipboard. Just as I turned in to the Day Room, I heard, 'Wait! *You*, there!'

I kept walking, thinking she was calling someone else.

'Wait, I say. *You*, girl!' She strode over to me. 'Who are you?'

'Judith Kruger.'

She dropped her eyes to the clipboard and checked off my name with a pencil stub.

'You came here while I was on leave. You don't know me and I don't know you. But we'll get along fine if you carry your own weight on this ward. Everyone pitches in here to keep A Ward clean. And no one loafs on my shift. Do you understand?'

'Yes, Miss Spence.'

'Now where were you going?'

'No place. I mean, over to my cabinet.'

She surveyed the Day Room and tapped the pencil against her teeth.

'Do you see those girls in there washing down the walls? Get a rag and go help them. I want this whole ward spick and span. Now get busy.'

I joined Beverly, Florence Adamski, and Esther. We talked very little. Each of us knew what the other was thinking. Once Beverly said, 'Do we need more water? This is dirty.' She stared sadly at the pail.

Esther stood up. 'Oh, my aching back! I'll get it.' She picked up the pail and jerked her thumb in the direction of Miss Spence, who was standing at the end of the Day Room like a boss supervising a work gang.

'Screw her', said Esther. 'From now until Christmas. While I'm filling this pail I'm going to grab a smoke. If she asks for me, tell her I dropped dead from overwork.'

Miss Spence went off duty at three. By three-thirty the tension had eased off. Beds began to fill up again. A student nurse unlocked the main bathroom. We crowded in for our first smoke since breakfast and traded invectives for Adelaide Spence. I stood in the corner, thinking of ways to—get lost as soldiers do in the Army. I don't think it should be too hard to learn the knack of quick disappearance when Miss Bastard hunts down her daily quota of forced labour. I'm not going to scrub another wall if I can help it.

My emotional control is still very ragged, susceptible to the slightest stimulus. Reading in my library book about a young child starting school, I thought with a quiver of panic, *how will Gary learn to read? To talk? To walk? How will he grow and*

8

develop? What must I do to help, to keep step with an ever-changing child? What are the rules and the signs?

I have to see Doctor Downey again as soon as I get home. It was stupid of me to resent him just because he didn't write me a letter. The stupidity of sickness. . . . My concentration broken, I read sporadically, skipping passages and flipping pages, barely understanding the story.

Then Nancy Kile screamed. She had been sitting a few feet away. Now she was standing up, her hands clutching the table, her eyes almost sightless, and her mouth hanging open. A bubbling guttural grunt came from her throat.

She scared me. I jumped up, banged the book down, and started to shake. A nurse and an attendant rushed over to Nancy. They pulled her hands from the table and pushed her down. Then they opened a colouring book and put a crayon in her hand.

'All right, Nancy. All right', the nurse said. 'Here's your book. Make pictures, Nancy. Pictures.' Nancy grinned and scratched the crayon across the page.

I went to the bathroom for a smoke but none of my friends was there. The only familiar face was that of Connie, still sitting on the toilet, rocking and scratching, her lips framing her when-I-go-home refrain.

Am getting fed up being cooped up. Am very restless. Maybe it's the heat. The air is heavy tonight. Smells sick. Wish it were time for bed. Very tired. Muscles ache from washing walls this morning. And tomorrow Miss Spence will be here and the damned hop-skip-and-jump will start again. Florence is playing the accordion. Can't make out the melody. Wonder if she takes request numbers? I'd like to hear 'Show Me the Way to Go Home'.

Tuesday, September 12

Feel better this morning. Joked with the girls in the cafeteria line. I like it when they laugh at my remarks. But I'm still functioning on two levels. Am lively and animated on the outside and nervous and tense inside. The rhymes and rhythms and sing-song patterns of thought still fill my head. Wonder if the doctors were right? Am I a manic-depressive? I'm swinging high now. Will I reach a peak and then fall?

Very anxious to go home again this week-end. Must keep testing myself in the home environment. Wish they had a system whereby patients could return home for a few weeks to gauge their own adjustment. No. It wouldn't work out. They'd lie to keep from coming back here. So would I. I'd have to panic again completely before I'd admit I wasn't ready for full release.

I live on the edge of hope. Like an animal, I pounce on each day and tear it to shreds. Then I dissect each little moment, each feeling of confidence or fear, and stack them in piles of pro and con, yes or no, better or worse, ready or not.

Wednesday, September 13

Doctor Manning has been interviewing since lunchtime and it's now almost two o'clock. The ward is tense and quiet. Patients are clustered in small tight groups. They whisper to each other. There is no laughter.

I've walked up and down the Day Room, through the corridors, and in and out of the washrooms. I see a hundred different faces, each with the same expression of muted fear and anticipation, each with eyes that mirror anxiety.

I'm too restless to join a group and listen to the chorus chanting 'do you think he'll get to me today?' . . . 'if I go to Staff' . . . 'they say that' . . . 'she's been in there a long time' . . . 'I had twenty shocks—I should go home' . . . 'there goes another one' . . . 'you look scared' . . . 'I'm not scared' . . . 'the hell you're not' . . . 'the longer he keeps you the better it is' . . . 'you sure?' . . . 'sure, I heard . . .'

Everybody talks and no one really knows. They make me nervous. Wish he'd call me and the whole thing were over. Wonder if he'll shoot questions like bullets to rattle me. Or maybe he'll just sit and stare and study me like a specimen. He'll see how my hands shake. Want to cut off these hands and stuff them in my pockets. How important he must feel, sitting at that desk, playing judge and jury. Passing sentences and granting reprieves. I hate him. Oh, this is no good. I'm working up a fury. They may call me any minute.

Well, it's over. A nurse called me when I was sitting outside on a bench. I ran up the steps smoothing my dress and hair, my heart pounding like a sledgehammer. He was sitting at that table with a pile of folders next to him. He was very tanned and his black eyes looked like coals in his head.

'Hello, Judith. Sit down.'

'Hello, Doctor Manning. Did you have a nice leave?' I stared at the ashtray.

'Fine. Well, how do you feel?'

'Good. Very good. Like my old self.'

Was that a good self?

'Are you still afraid of your baby?'

'Oh, no.'

Not much. Only very much.

'Do you feel competent to handle him?'

'Yes. I did very well last week-end. And my mother will stay with me. I want to start therapy again when I get home. I need more help. I——'

'Definitely. We expect you to continue therapy.'

'Oh, I will. I will.'

'Well, you seem in pretty fair shape. I don't think you'll be here too long. I'll check with Doctor Heineman, but I think we'll take you off shock. All right. You can go now.'

'Thank you, Doctor Manning. Thanks a lot.'

Why doesn't he smile? Isn't he happy for me? Isn't he glad I'm recovering? I want to say so much, but his face won't let me.

I started to open the door, but my hands were dripping with sweat and the knob wouldn't turn. (*Quick! Get out before he changes his mind.*) I wrenched the door open and turned to him. 'Doctor Manning, I want to thank you for——'

He waved his hand at me. 'For a while there I thought surely you'd blow up in complete panic!'

'Oh, but I'm better now. So much better.' I forced a big smile and ran out into the hall.

Why did he have to say that? Why did he turn the screw? To sober me and keep me in line? He didn't have to remind me. I'll remember. *And how* I'll remember!

Back in the Day Room, Bertha motioned me over. Beverly was sitting with her.

'Look', Bertha said. 'I got a letter from Laura. She's still resting up. She says she misses the girls and the card games. She sent you a special regard. Here. Read this.'

Laura's script was thick and up-slanted. At the bottom of the page she had written, 'Tell Judith I miss her jokes and the funny way she plays cards. I pray for you, all of you, every day. May God make you whole again and let you return to your loved ones.'

'That's very nice of her', I said. 'When you write again, please send her my best wishes.'

'I pray every day, too', Beverly said. Her eyes were large and moist. 'Today I'm praying extra hard for the interview. You saw him, didn't you, Judith?'

'Yes. I just came out of there.'

They both leaned forward, and Bertha said, 'Well, is it a secret? What did he say?'

'He said I'm doing pretty well and I won't be here long. He didn't mention a date, but——'

'Wonderful', Bertha chuckled. She squeezed my hand. 'I'm so glad for you.'

'Me too', Beverly said. But her face looked long and drawn. 'What about shock?'

'He doesn't think they'll give me any more.'

'Boy, are you ever the worrier!' Bertha said. She slapped at the air with her hand. 'All that fuss about the letter that day! Remember?'

'I hope they stop shock for me too', Beverly said. 'I had just as many as you did.'

'I hope so, too. I hope both of you get good news.'

I really do. I like you. You have been nice to me, You didn't chase me away when I was so upset. You are my friends here. But I don't know what's wrong with you. This isn't a game of cards where each player has an equal chance to win freedom.

'They took Connie away a few minutes ago', Beverly said.

'No! You mean she did go home? After all that talking?'

'No,' Bertha said, 'they transferred her to another ward. It's better if you stay here in A Ward. This is an active treatment ward. Lots of patients go home from here.'

'I wish you'd had your interviews, Bev and Bertha. Are you afraid? I was.'

'No', Bertha said. 'Why should I be afraid?' She dropped her eyes to the deck of cards on the table and scooped them up in her short, fat hands. 'Who wants to play bridge?'

'A little later. Thanks.' I wanted to be alone right now, to recapitulate the interview and savour the good parts.

Two new patients were sprawled on my bed. I grew hot with rage.

Why can't they keep off other people's property? I don't like people touching my things. They've mussed up the spread. I bet it's all dirty.

'Hello', I said.

'What do *you* want?' one of them answered.

I tightened inside. More nasty ones. Why are some so nasty when they're sick? I was sick, but I was nice and polite.

'I'd like to sit on my bed. Do you mind?'

'It ain't your bed. It's the hospital's', the other one said.

'I sleep here, so it's my bed. Should I find the nurse? She'll tell you it's my bed.' I knew she'd scoot us all out of there, but I couldn't resist the threat. I don't know why, but I wanted to fight. I felt my hands clench into fists and the blood run hot in my face.

'Come on', said the first. 'Leave the bitch alone.' As they walked away, she stuck out her tongue at me.

'Go to hell', I shouted.

I wonder what got into me? I've had run-ins before with anti-social patients, but I've always retreated. This time I spoke as I felt. It's a new thing for me.

Tonight they had games in the Auditorium.

The place looked so different from the last time I was there. Most of the seats on the main floor were cleared away. Shuffle-board markings were painted on the floor. There were ping-pong tables and card tables stacked with draughts and cards.

But the big room looked empty. There were only twenty or thirty people there, most of them sitting on benches along the wall. They looked so ill at ease. The women patients were clustered on one side and the men on the other.

Male and female nurses kept walking up and down trying to coax us to start some games. I was annoyed with the women. I wanted so much to join a game. It was good to be there, to see the men again. For an instant, I felt as I had at my first high school dance, sitting with giggling and whispering girls secretly ogling the boys across the room. So young and yet so grown. Hair slicked down. Shirt collars cutting into their necks. Restless. Shifting from one foot to the other. Fidgeting with ties and pocket handkerchiefs, casting quick glances at our rustling skirts, our flipping curls, and the toes of our pointed party shoes.

I turned to the women from my ward. 'Well, who's going to break the ice? Esther? Helen? Bev? You want to play ping-pong? It's a shame to come here and then just sit around like this. Come on!'

Then I saw the fellow who had sat next to me at the concert. He was sitting on the apron of the empty stage tossing a ping-pong ball in the air. I broke away from the women and walked to him. Again I had the feeling I was fourteen years old. My cheeks were burning and my throat dry.

'Say, how about throwing the ball at me? I mean, across the ping-pong table?'

This is a man, my mind hummed. His very maleness demands that I parade myself and my personality and win him over.

He caught the ball and closed both hands over it. I thought he would crush it. *Answer me, please*, I begged inside. Don't make me go back there alone. They'll laugh at my boldness and failure. You can't be very sick or they wouldn't have brought you here tonight.

Finally he stood up, nodded his head, and handed me the ball. As he reached across the table for the racquets I saw a slow red flush suffuse his neck. Patches of perspiration had darkened the underarms of his faded blue shirt.

He's nervous, I thought. And so am I. Maybe he's afraid of me. I forced him into this. I'm sorry.

'Will you serve or should I?'

'O.K.', he said.

'O.K., what?' I tried to laugh. 'Me or you?'

He threw the ball to me, but his aim was poor. I had to chase it. When I came back he said, 'I'm sorry.'

'That's O.K. Ready?' And then I forgot about him. I was caught in the thrill of the game. All my pent-up energy spilled out in a fury of slashing and slamming at the ball. He was a poor player. His serves were weak and he hit into the net. But I didn't care. I ran after the balls, called out the score, and chattered away. 'Oh, that was a good one. . . . A little closer and it would have been in. . . . Your serve, right? . . . Oh, you're doing fine . . .'

. I slammed the ball off the edge of the table. 'My game. Thanks. That was fun. Want to play another?'

He nodded and turned to a man standing nearby. 'Joe, want a game?' he asked.

'O.K.,' Joe said.

I spoke to my partner. 'I don't know your name. I'm Judith.'

'Larry', he said.

'Larry, Joe, Judith', I said, and pointed to each of us like a you-Tarzan-me-Jane routine. 'Wait. We need another one for doubles. Beverly!' I called. 'Come on. We need you.'

She shook her head at me from the bench. I ran to her. 'Bev, it's fun.'

'But I can't——'

'But, but, but! Come on!' I pulled her up, pushed her to the table, and shoved a racquet into her hand. It was ice cold. 'Beverly, you and Joe against Larry and me. O.K.?'

'I don't play good.' Her eyes were begging, pleading, but I felt no pity.

'So what? It's just for the hell of it.' I ran round the table, almost pushing them into their positions.

The game was a hodge-podge of 'Oops, sorry . . . Your point? . . . Who serves? . . . What's the score? . . . I chased the balls. I fixed the net when it fell down. I ran myself ragged to keep the game going. We had almost finished two games when a male nurse came over and told the men it was time to go. They laid the racquets on the table and walked after the nurse. They didn't wave to us or make any gesture of good-bye.

'I'm tired', Beverly said.

'So am I', I answered. And I was. Physically and emotionally. I had acted like a one-woman Y.W.C.A. But I can't help it. The sight of people together throws me into a violent discharge of words and action. I must organize and galvanize. Pump laughter and life into the party. Talk and keep talking and never relax. Never drop the mask of hilarity or they will see you naked and empty and you will have lost them.

Thursday, September 14

Something's wrong with Bertha. When I came back to the ward last night she was crying. The girls told me she'd been crying since five o'clock, after her interview with Doctor Manning. Today her face is puffy and blotched and her eyes are red-rimmed. This morning I said, 'Please, Bertie. Let me help you. You helped me. We're friends, Bertha. Talk to me. Remember when I came? I kept telling everyone how sick I was. And you listened and you helped me. Can't I do the same for you? Please, Bertha?'

She ground her fat hands into her eyes. 'There's nothing you can do.' Her voice was flat and dead. 'It's too late.'

'What's too late?'

'Everything. Nothing. Please leave me alone.'

Friday, September 15

The ward seems more crowded each day. I don't like the new ones. They're strangers, usurpers, crowding us out of our cafeteria seats, our beds, and our smoking places in the washrooms. I know this is nonsense. This place isn't a private sorority house or a country club. No one voluntarily applies for membership here! Yet I think of Laura and the lonely look in her eyes when she said good-bye. Then I had thought, *poor girl, she's really not well yet. How can she be so reluctant to leave a mental hospital?*

Now I think I understand. Familiarity turns the bitter to the sweet. And day by day the world within the walls becomes more comforting than the world without.

I had judged Laura in the heat of fear. Tonight, if she were here, I would sit with her. We would talk about music and books. We would play some cards. We would eat our fruit and candy. We would watch the night creep through the windows and share a silent understanding.

Mrs. Matthews just pattered over to me. 'Thought you'd like to know, Judith. You've got another week-end pass. I just came on duty and saw it on the board.'

'Thanks, Mrs. Matthews', I said. 'Thanks a lot. I'm off shock now. You know?'

'Yes, I know. Have a good time, huh?'

Maybe it will be good. I have to try and keep trying. I can't hide here for ever.

Sunday night, September 17

Jay stepped off the lift on Saturday at the stroke of nine.

'Hello, Rock of Gibraltar', I said.

'Hello, sweetie. How are you? Say, what do you mean, Rock of Gibraltar?'

'You're so prompt. I can always count on you.'

'Would you want me to come at noon?'

'Oh, no. I'm glad you're here early. I appreciate it. Really I do.'

What was I trying to say? That I'm jealous of him? That I resent the fact I can't find fault?

We were standing by the lift when Beverly came running up. Her sallow face was flushed. 'Judith, I'm going home for Sunday. I saw Doctor Manning yesterday. I prayed I wouldn't be nervous. But I was. It's all right, though. He said they'll stop shock soon. He——' Her face lost its animation and she shrank again. 'Hello, Jay', she said. 'Judith's told me a lot about you.'

'Has she?'

'Jay, this is my friend Beverly.'

'You're very nice. You look like a doctor.' There was awe in her eyes.

'Thank you, Beverly.'

Suddenly I hated him. He sounded so professional and patronizing. Is that how he talks to his patients? As if he's talking to a child? Maybe that's how he feels towards me. A sick little girl who needs calm and careful handling lest she go into a tantrum again.

When we stepped into the lift Beverly waved, a little hesitant, a little brave. 'Have a good time. Kiss Gary for me.'

'I will,' I called back, 'and thanks.'

I didn't speak until we were well on the highway.

'I saw Doctor Manning this week.'

'What did he say?'

'That I won't be here much longer. That I'm in pretty good shape.'

'Good!' He took his hand from the wheel and squeezed mine. His eyes looked happy. 'I love you, sweetie. I'm so glad you're getting better.'

'He asked me how I felt about the baby. If I was still frightened of him. I told him I think I could handle it now.'

'I think you can, too.'

'I don't. I blow hot and cold. Some days I'm fine. Other times I think of him and I get scared. Very scared. That's when I'd rather stay in the hospital.'

'Sweetie, you'll have those feelings for a while. It's normal.'

'Normal for the abnormal, huh?'

'You're not abnormal.'

'Oh, no! I had a baby and fell apart—that's all! There's not a thing wrong with me.'

'Stop knocking yourself. Thousands of women have depressions.'

'I'm not thousands of women. I'm me. And I hate myself. Oh, Jay, I almost forgot. Did you come to the hospital to talk to the doctors?'

'Yes. This past Wednesday.'

'What happened?'

'Nothing much. They asked me a few questions about you. How you were when you were well. In that letter you sent me you kept using the words manic-depressive. Is that what you're afraid of?'

'Yes. That Doctor Connor put a bug in my ear.'

'Well, you're not. And they know it, too. You're coming along fine. You're getting well.' His hand touched my thigh. I remembered that morning, so long ago, when I had begged him to caress me, to stave off the creeping numbness of body and mind. Then it was no good. But now I was alive again, and the pressure of his fingers made me tremble. . . .

The week-end was the same as the last. My hands and eyes were never still. I tried to take on every responsibility. A nappy is soiled? Quick, rinse it out. . . . A spoon and a cup in the sink? Wash them. . . . Run to the line in the yard, pull off Gary's shirt and put it away. . . . Jay's towel is hanging bunched on the rack. Smooth it out. . . . Is that dust on the windowsill? Grab a rag and wipe it away. . . . Order, order, everything come to order. The only things I couldn't touch were my clothes. I am still afraid of them.

On Sunday afternoon I was sitting on the back steps when I heard a sound behind me.

'Oh, Jay. You startled me. I don't hear you coming when you wear those hospital shoes.'

'How are you doing, darling?'

'Fine. A little tired.'

'I'll be off duty at five. Would you want to take a walk? We don't have to start back until after six.'

'No. If you don't mind.'

Scared to walk a street. To see merchandise in store windows, film marquees, parents pushing baby carriages, all the signs and symbols of living and doing and being. It still hurts. The wound of fear is still not healed. I'm a freak and a misfit. I've run from the world and the flesh of my flesh. So they put me in a hospital. They gave me shock to stop me from running and turn me round in the right direction. And now they're all waiting to see how far I've returned. Jay is waiting. And my parents. And Gary is waiting, too, although he doesn't know it. They are holding out their arms to me, in a circle of support. But the circle looks like a trap.

We were driving back to the hospital. The sun was low and fingers of twilight crept from the East.

'Sweetie,' he said, 'you didn't seem as happy this time. You were restless and nervous.'

'I'm always that way. And I don't know what it is to be happy. So that's no criterion.'

'You're still afraid to come home?'

'Yes. I'm not in panic any more. And I'm not depressed. But I don't know what I want. I know what I *should* want and how I *ought* to feel, but that's no good. What's wrong with me?'

'I don't know.' He clicked on the headlights. It was almost dark.

'Are you lying to me? You're a doctor.'

'But I'm not a psychiatrist. Even if I were, it wouldn't help much. You're not a patient. You're my wife.'

'Are you sorry I'm your wife? I'm not much good now.'

'Don't be silly. You will be. You are getting better. You're afraid to believe it, aren't you?'

'Yes.'

The gates of the hospital were up ahead. Night sounds filtered through the open car window. Crickets sang by the side of the road. A solitary bird warbled high in a tree. Then our tyres crunched on the gravel road and the cluster of hospital buildings loomed against the new night sky.

'Stop the car a minute.'

He glanced at his watch. 'O.K. We have a little time.'

I reached for his hand and slipped my fingers through his. He leaned over and kissed my cheek. 'Nice night for necking, huh? We used to do a lot of it, remember? But not in the car.'

'No,' I answered. 'Central Park, Bronx Park, Van Cortlandt Park.'

'All the parks.' His fingers traced a pattern on my arm.

'The benches were hard.'

'We got the car too late. We were married then.'

'Then we had a bed. Remember how it creaked? We always thought the landlady could hear us.' He squeezed my shoulder. 'We had fun, didn't we?'

'Uh-huh. There's no fun now, is there?'

'I guess not. But it'll come.'

'I've made a mess of things, Jay.'

'It's not your fault. Don't blame yourself.'

'Who do I blame, then? My mother? My father?'

'Could be. Anything could be.'

'Now that's silly. I just mentioned their names. The first names I thought of. I could have said the man in the moon.'

'They're much closer to you than the moon.'

'You don't like them, do you? You always pick on them.'

'And you're always protecting them against imaginary attacks. I never said I don't like them.'

'Don't you appreciate what they're doing for me?'

'Of course I appreciate it.'

You do like hell. You take for granted everything they give. I can never repay them for their sacrifices. And you, you have no feelings of obligation. I hate you for that.

'Judy, we'd better go in now. It's twenty to eight.'

He drove the car into the puddle of light in front of Ward A building.

'Sweetie, I wish we were coming home now. Together.'

Tears clouded my eyes. 'I'm sorry. I keep giving you a hard time. I don't know why.'   :

'When you start treatment you'll find out. The acute stage is over. You'll be seeing things more clearly. You'll be able to dig to the roots.'

'That's what I'm afraid of.'

'There's nothing fearful in finding out about yourself. It's important and it's good.' He opened the car door and helped me out. I shivered in the cool night air. I saw a nurse leaning in the doorway, silhouetted in the light from the lobby.

'I feel like a commuter.' I pointed to her. 'There's the conductor waiting to punch my pass.'

He laughed. 'Maybe next time it'll be a one-way trip home. Would you like that?'

'I think so—I hope so. Maybe you're right. I'm just afraid to believe I'm getting well.'

As the nurse closed the lift door I saw him standing there and smiling. It wasn't a big smile, wide and grinny. But I knew he was telling me '*I love you. Keep trying.*'

Monday, September 18

Last night I expected to lie awake for hours, reliving the week-end. Instead, a strange leaden calm settled over me. I could only remember Jay's face smiling as I stood in the lift. His strength and love, that which I've clutched at and rejected, only to reach for again, blocked out all the little fears.

I woke early and went to the small bathroom. It was crowded with patients and the clock read only ten to six. A woman bent over the basin straightened up and blinked away the water. I squinted at her. It was Bertha.

'Bertha! What are you doing here? You sleep in the big ward.'

'They changed my bed.' Her fat face was impassive.

'Why?'

'I'm on insulin. Starting today.'

'You're joking!'

'I'm not joking.' She reached for the towel jammed between her knees and wiped her face and hands.

Mrs. Hendricks bustled in. 'Now hurry up, girls. You have to be back in bed by six. Come on, Bertha . . . Margaret . . . you there . . . little blondie . . . are you ready?' She pushed through the crowded room patting shoulders and buttocks.

Then she saw me. 'Judith, dearie. What are you doing here? Get back to your ward.' She grabbed my wrist and whispered to me, 'These are insulin patients, honey. First day, you know? Some are a little fretty. Now run along like a good girl.'

When she left I edged back to Bertha. I was bursting with questions. But she was staring straight ahead, her eyes empty, smoothing down the front of her nightgown.

'Bertie, I'm . . . I'm sorry.'

'There's nothing to be sorry for.' She didn't look at me. 'It's not your fault. It's not anybody's.' And then she blinked her eyes. 'I wish Laura was here. I don't know any of these women. Just her.' She pointed to the corner of the room.

'Who's that?' I couldn't see.

'Your friend Mary. She whined all last night when she heard she was going on insulin.'

'How do you feel, Bertha?' My voice came out all wrong. It sounded morbid and unctuous. I should have left. But I was waiting for her to tell me what had happened with that interview with Doctor Manning.

'I feel lousy.'

'Maybe it'll be just a few treatments.'

'No. I'm getting the full course. Twenty.'

'Gee, I'm sorry. I——'

'Stop saying that.'

'I think I'd better go.'

'Yeah, you'd better.'

I pushed my way to the door. 'I'll see you later, Bertha. Good luck.'

She didn't answer.

At nine-thirty the Day Room was almost empty. The doors to the insulin wards had been shut since six o'clock. And now the electro-shock patients had gone into the big ward to undress. I sat by a table, fingering a deck of cards. I kept thinking of Bertha. How she used to sit here in her neat cotton print dress, her hair set and wrapped in a bright kerchief, and her big voice booming with laughter. Now I was alone. I felt strangely out of place, living on the fringes of A Ward routine. For the first time, I looked forward to Miss Spence stalking through the Day Room to pick up her strays for clean-up. I looked up, half expecting to see her. Then Doctor Manning came walking down the aisle. I jumped up.

'Doctor Manning, could I speak to you for a moment?'

Always tell them a moment or a second. Let them know you appreciate how rushed they are.

'Yes?'

'I'm feeling quite well. I was wondering if I could get more O.T. Maybe in the mornings, too. I like it. I like to keep busy.'

'I've put you up for Staff tomorrow, Judith.'

I was so surprised I stuttered. 'S-s-staff?'

'Yes. Wait until then. We'll see how it goes. I think you'll pass.' He smiled, his teeth white against his tanned face.

'Oh. Yes. Thank you. Thanks a million. I really appreciate it.'

The smile was gone. 'You know we rarely let a patient go to Staff so soon. But you've come round pretty well. And of course you're starting psychotherapy as soon as you get home, aren't you?'

'Oh, definitely. Right away.'

Sooner than soon, Doctor. The very instant.

He strode away. I didn't move until he unlocked the door to the shock ward and disappeared inside. Then I sat down in a heap, flooded with excitement. Staff, Staff, Staff. The word beat in my brain. Up for Staff. Up from the depths. Placed on a platter for perusal by the gods. Prisoner in a box. Interrogation and judgment. Sentence pronounced. Free. Or remanded back to custody. If you make it, you stand up and walk out. If you fall, you sink down again and back to the end of the line.

But I'll make it, I told myself. Staff is an examination. I've always been good at exams. They'll test me in a way I can handle. They'll watch how I sit, what I do with my hands. They'll listen to my voice and how I frame answers to their questions. I'll be on display. I don't mind that. It's a challenge I can meet. When I step into that Staff room I'll be on a stage. I'll play a role that will win them over. *He thinks I'm well enough for Staff!* That's all I need to know.

My chest was bursting with excitement. I felt like a student again, anticipating end of term. My final in Mental Health. If I pass, I'll be graduated. Wonder if this place gives diplomas? I laughed inside.

Tuesday, September 19

They'll come for me any minute now. Feel so dressed up. I went to Millie to ask for a clean dress for my storage bin.

'Ain't you goin' to change your shoes, too? Those moccasins you're wearin' are beat. Here's a nice pair of shoes.' She was standing on a stool and peering into my clothes bin. 'New red ones. Put 'em on.'

'No, wait. This dress is green. Isn't there a pair of green and yellow shoes up there?'

'Yeah. Here they are. Way in the back.' She handed them down to me. 'And here's a pretty slip. Put that on, too. You hear?' She hopped off the stool. 'Now go get dressed. Then I wanna see you. I wanna see that you did yourself right.'

'Thanks, Millie. You've been nice to me.'

'Hell, you ain't goin' yet. You're just goin' up to Staff, girl.' She locked the closet door. 'Now fix yourself up. You wanna look nice for the doctors.' She slapped me on the behind. 'Beats me how you usta wear those state clothes!'

I went back to the main washroom. Every week it was some-one else who drew a circle round her with the mention of Staff. Someone else who stepped from anonymity into a barrage of encouragement tinged with envy; who primped and fussed and came to the washroom clique for approval and advice.

'. . . Now, look, don't be nervous. It's no good if you're nervous . . . smile . . . my friend told me you should always smile . . . no, don't smile. Be quiet. You know . . . reserved . . . just answer their questions . . . I tell you you ought to . . . now do like I say . . . listen to me . . . '

I used to stand apart from these huddles. I didn't know what they meant by Staff and I didn't care. As I came out of the depression I drew towards them, slowly, cautiously, and listened to the words of warning, trying to store up scraps of information. Now it was my turn. But I couldn't show them how happy I was. I couldn't crow. Behind the smiles, behind the awe in the

9

eyes of new patients, I knew they were thinking, *if only it were me instead of her! When will I go? When? WHEN?*

This took the edge off my excitement. I watched them staring at me and I felt embarrassed that I had been chosen for a chance at freedom. And yet there are only a few I like here. Most of them are strangers who break my sleep with screams, who corner me with blazing eyes and tales of persecution, or cut me with silence when I try to make conversation.

This is not a happy place. We don't make fast friendships here. We don't sign our names in autograph books and pledge ourselves to remember until Niagara Falls. We don't arrange future dates and family visits. We spin each in her own orbit. Some keep spinning. Some break through. And when we break, we run. We don't look back.

3 p.m. ·

Since lunchtime they have been chanting at me, singly, or in groups, 'Did'ja pass, did'ja pass, did'ja pass?'

I shrug my shoulders and smile. 'I don't know. I think so. I don't know.'

'How wuzzit, how wuzzit, how wuzzit?' the chorus asks.

I give them a quick nod of the head. 'Pretty good. Not hard.'

'Whadid they askyou, whadid they askyou?' the voices rise.

'Some questions. Not many. A few questions', I reply. Then I stop the music with 'every case is different', my palms up and open in apology that I cannot tell them more. I remember Laura. I had thought she was unduly evasive when I pressed her for details after her Staff conference. Now I understand.

They're busy now, sitting out here on the benches and grass. I think they're through with me. Now I can mull the thing over; savour it with private pleasure. . . . It went well. Very well. When the student nurse came for me I looked at my hands. They were still and calm. That was a good sign.

'Am I the only one from Ward A today?' I asked her.

'Yes. There aren't too many hold-overs from the summer. Therapy's started again, you know.'

'Yes.' I thought of Bertha in the insulin ward.

'You nervous?'

'No. I feel good. I was more nervous about getting shock

treatments. I hated them. I—(*Wrong to say that. You're not safe yet. Don't talk so freely. She's just liable to——*) I mean at first. They helped me. They really did.'

When we stepped off the lift I recognized the Admissions ward immediately. Was it only seven weeks ago that I lay in that big room over there wrapped in terror? I saw the fat old Negro woman lumber past. She was still wearing the same stocking cap on her head. I thought, probably on her way to beg a glass of juice for another new admission.

'Wait here a minute. I have to pick up another one.' She left me in the hall opposite the office where I first saw Doctor Manning. It was empty now. Sunlight was streaming on the desk and chairs. But I could still see him as he looked that night, his legs crossed high, his eyes appraising me as I pleaded for a transfer. And I heard myself crying and begging, struggling for coherence from a mind disorganized with fear and depression. My cheeks flushed hot with shame. But I knew that if ever I had a relapse I would be as helpless to control myself as I had been that night. When you are suffocating, there is no time for reason and decorum. You yell for help.

'O.K., let's go.' The nurse was back with a middle-aged woman walking next to her. 'Letty, this is Judith', she said.

'Hello. How are you, Letty?' I spoke up bright and friendly.

She didn't answer me. She wound a strand of straggling grey hair round her ear and wiped her hands on the front of a dirty cotton dress.

What the hell's the matter with her? She's going to Staff. She's being considered for release. And she won't even say hello. Look at her. So messy and dirty. In my ward we shower and change into our best dresses. We set our hair and put on fresh make-up and spray ourselves with cologne. And this one! Bet she passes, too!

We crossed the ward and took another lift ride and came off into a large waiting-room. I remembered this floor. We passed through here on the way for our spinals. From the adjoining offices the click-clack of typewriters punched the air.

Funny, I thought. Or is it? Only a few months ago I had a desk in an office and banged on my typewriter like that. Now I sit here in a mental hospital, waiting for my release.

About half a dozen patients were scattered on the benches.

The nurse from my ward and two others stood to one side, holding case-history folders. Directly opposite the benches was a green door on which was lettered the word 'STAFF'.

White-coated technicians passed by. Orderlies wheeled equipment trays on and off the lift. Secretaries minced along on high-heeled polished pumps, their heels clattering on the cement floor.

It's like Grand Central Station. We are sitting in the waiting-room. Waiting for a ticket to freedom. We carry no luggage. Just hope. Our minds and bodies are filled with it, breathing it, screaming with it. We don't talk. But when our eyes meet we smile a tight fleeting smile to acknowledge our mutual journey. Some of us fidget and squirm. Others sit quietly, hands folded in our laps. One of us is biting her nails.

It was I. The waiting made me restless. I wanted to walk round or talk to the nurses, to do something active. The tension was building. I ran my fingers along the slats of the bench. I crossed my legs and then uncrossed them. I smoothed the front of my dress.

Creased already. Hate it when dresses get creased, get dirty. Want them clean. Ready to wear but not to wear. Afraid to touch. Oh, God. Felt like this two months ago. Now it's come back. Why now? I'm better. I know I'm better. Just getting a little nervous, that's all.

I went over to my nurse. 'Excuse me, I was just wondering. They take us in turn, don't they? I mean, those other women, they're all ahead of me?'

'Yes. Impatient?'

'A little.'

'Once they start, it goes pretty fast. There! They've opened the door. Now go and sit down. It won't be long.'

When a nurse came out of the Staff room we sat up straight and tall, as grade-school children do when the teacher comes into the room. She didn't look at us. She took the folders from the student nurses, walked back to the Staff door, opened the first folder, and called out, 'Djendjielewski!'

A tiny blonde woman popped from her seat like a jack-in-the box. What a name, I laughed inside. She'll be out in a minute. They'll ask her just one question: Spell and pronounce your name. If she does that, she's ready for anything.

I'm silly. I'm making fun of things. Playing with absurdities. Looking for relief in ridicule. Relax. Look out of the window. Count the flowers on your dress. And the tiles on the wall. Get your mind away from that Staff door.

The door opened and the little blonde came out. The nurse called another name. The student nurse was right. It doesn't take long. Then another name, and another. Then——

'Kruger.'

'Here!' I moved to the door. My heart was pounding.

Weren't going to be frightened, were you? Would be a cinch, remember? And now you're hot and cold. There's a hole where your stomach should be and your tongue is thick and dry and burning.

'Over here, Judith. On that chair.' I had been staring at the green rug under my feet until I eased into the chair. Then I looked up. The room was filled with doctors. They were sitting two and three deep behind a long mahogany table.

Is this the Staff? It looks like a medical convention!

'Good morning, Judith.'

Who's talking? So many I can't tell.

'Good morning.' I spoke to the far end of the table, my eyes trying to locate the voice.

'How are you feeling?'

'Well. Pretty well.'

Got the adverb right, didn't you? Now if I could just see who—— There she is. Big grey-haired woman. Hair piled on her head. Big brooch on her dress. Nice face. Motherly. Looks like someone I knew.

'Do you think you're ready to go home?'

Doctor Manning. There on the left. No smile. No sign. Nothing to show he's my doctor.

'Yes. I think so.'

Easy now. Your hands. Relax them. And look at him. Your head a little to one side, your face composed in polite attention. The little tricks. Remember?

'Are you still afraid of the baby?' he asked.

'No. I've come to accept him. I'm more at ease. I enjoy taking care of him now. When I've gone home it felt good to see him and hold him.'

O.K. Cut it. The more you say, the more chance for a blunder.

'Who's taking care of your baby?'

The woman again. Now I know. My art teacher in Junior High. The spit'n' image.

'My mother. She's living with me.'

'And she'll stay on?'

'Oh, yes. As long as I need her.'

'You went to college, didn't you?'

'Yes.'

'What was your major?'

'Home Economics.'

'Well,' she plumped in the chair and smiled, 'I don't think you'll have too much trouble with the house and baby care.'

Silly. She means well, but so silly. Doesn't know how little I was suited for Home Economics. Don't answer. Just smile. Wait for the others to talk. I see Doctor Heineman. He ought to be good for a question or two. Well? Why are they staring? I'm not a freak, am I? Watch it now. Hold that half-smile, that sweet expression. Don't get rattled.

'I understand you'll start therapy as soon as you're home?' The woman again.

'Yes. Right away. I already have a doctor.'

'Well, I think that will be all for now. Unless there are any more questions?' She turned to the others. There was no response. 'We'll notify your husband. Good luck to you, Judith.'

'Thank you. Thank you very much.'

Get up slowly. Don't push the chair. There's the nurse coming for you. She was waiting by the door all the time. Follow her out. Don't look back. You'll have to say thank you again. Few steps more. Door open now. Door closed. Now breathe. Deep. It's over. It's all over.

8.30 p.m.

What are they trying to do to me? Am so frightened I can't hold this pencil steady. Until twenty minutes ago the day had been so good, so very good.

I know I passed Staff. That woman doctor said they'll notify Jay. And she wished me good luck. I know what that means. Any day now ... any day ... over the hump ... up and over ... I chanted and chattered to myself. The hours flew by. I watched television after supper and laughed. Then I smoked a final cigarette and looked out of the window in the washroom. The pine trees were straight and beautiful against the night sky.

It's cool tonight, I thought. Good for sleeping. Think I'll take two blankets. My ward is cold in the morning. I was rummaging through the bundles of nightgowns looking for my name stick when Mrs. Matthews came in.

'Judith? You here?'

'Yes.' I straightened up. 'Here I am.'

'We've had to rearrange the beds. You'll sleep in the main ward tonight.'

'All right. Which bed, Mrs. Matthews?'

'Second from the door on the left.' She walked out. I was a little disturbed at the change. Just when I get used to a spot they shift me around. It's all these new patients.

'Psst.' Beverly slithered into the room. She must have been just outside. All day long she had looked at me with happiness and envy. Now her eyes were different. They were wide and frightened.

'What's the matter, Beverly?'

'I heard her tell you they changed your bed. Do you know where you're sleeping? Do you know who's next to you?'

'No, and why all the whispering? What's wrong?'

'It's Josephine Hunter. You know. The big one. The one who curses. The one——'

I rushed past her and ran into the nursing office.

'Mrs. Matthews, could I sleep somewhere else tonight? Anywhere else?'

'Why?'

'I . . . I . . . I'm a little afraid of Josephine Hunter. That bed you assigned me. It's next to hers.'

'She won't bother you.'

'Can't I change? Please?'

'Nope. Not tonight. Look. Stop worrying. Don't talk to her. Go about your business and get into bed. I told you she won't bother you.' She swivelled in the chair and picked up a magazine.

Damn you. Damn you. You sit there on your fat behind and tell me not to worry. You won't sleep next to her, will you? Your guts won't turn to jelly as she sits in her bed, not two feet away from you, the hairy stubbles on her chin joggling up and down as she works her mouth in soundless monologues of hate.

Josephine's got her legs crossed now, and her arms are hanging ape-like from the sleeves of her nightgown. I'd better not look again. She may think I'm staring. Yet I can't turn my back. She may lunge at me in a sudden fury. My body feels huge. Every part of me is prickling with fear. Maybe I should stop writing before she thinks I'm a spy.

Bev passed by my bed a moment ago. I waved her away with flicking fingers. The nurse just came in to shut off the lights. Good night. Sweet dreams. Oh, God, I'm scared.

Wednesday, September 20

I woke this morning embarrassed that I had fallen asleep in spite of myself. I got up twice to go to the bathroom. Each time I looked at the huddled figure in the next bed I felt a new stab of fear. But it wasn't enough to keep me awake. It's funny and ironic. I can drop off to sleep in the presence of a physical fear. Yet tiny unrealities are strong enough to keep my brain racing through a sleepless night. It's always the little things with me. The gnawing things. The maybes and the yet-to-bes.

Well, this is September. I've spent the summer in a Pennsylvania country place.

'Have a good time?'

'Let's say it was different.'

'What about the food?'

'Adequate. Can't complain. Plain cooking.'

'And the guests? Meet any nice people?'

'They are all nice people. At least they were. You know how it is when you're taken away. I mean, get away from home.'

'Place crowded?'

'Very. New ones come every day.'

'How about the grounds?'

'Very lovely. Beautiful lawns and trees. I didn't get around much, though.'

'Nice activities for the guests?'

'Mostly indoor sports. Cards, puzzles, books, television, and talk. Plenty of talk.'

'Stimulating conversation, huh? Real intellectual?'

'No. More psychological than anything.'

'Well, that doesn't sound too bad. Coming back next year?'

'*No. Definitely not. Once is enough. It's no good to get too attached to a place.*'

As soon as breakfast was over I grabbed a mop and a pail and cleaned up the two small washrooms off the nursing corridor. I spent all morning there, working with deliberate slowness. I wanted the nurses to see me. Perhaps there was a memo lying on the office desk with word of the outcome of my Staff conference. Seeing me would jog their minds. Or maybe it was a telephone call taken and never jotted down. Something. Anything. I was so anxious. I even mopped the corridor in front of the lift. Each time the cables whined, I thought, *maybe the next one off will have some word for me*. It was a wasted morning. Except for Miss Spence, of course. She saw me sloshing the mop with a vigour I had never shown, trotted over and said crisply, like an Army colonel, 'Good job there, girl, good job.'

On the way to the cafeteria for lunch I saw Bertha sitting in the Day Room with the insulin patients. She was eating the late breakfast provided for them. They have to start insulin shock on empty stomachs.

I waved to her. She nodded briefly and turned back to the woman next to her, bending her head in private conversation. Since she's been on treatment, I haven't spoken ten words to her. She's drifted from me, intentionally or accidentally. There's a veil between us. She makes no attempt to maintain a friendship that was active and urgent only a few days ago.

I walked away, asking myself, what's happened to us? Do you suddenly hate me because you have to take treatment and I am finished? Bertha, we were as close as people can be in a place like this. Remember the jokes at cards, the smokes after meals, the way we sought out each other? And then you cried and cried and never told me why. And now you don't eat with me or talk with me. You sit with the new ones. Why?

This is silly. I am only days away from release and I can't get her out of my mind. Yet I know this is nothing new. I've felt this way before. If someone offers herself to me, I must return the relationship in double measure. Somehow it is my fault if they falter and slacken attention and drift away. I always blame myself for failure. Any kind of failure.

I like to watch Miss Willems when she comes on duty at three o'clock, her uniform is so white against her cream-brown skin. And each day she tucks yet another bright-coloured handkerchief in her breast pocket. I wait impatiently for her to approach me, for just the right moment to say hello. But today she stopped to talk with some new patients a few tables away. I riffled through a magazine. Still she didn't come. When she sat down with those patients, I grew angry. Then she touched one of them on the arm and smiled, the same soft smile she gave to me those first few days. I could feel the flush of jealousy in my face. I scraped back the chair and stamped to the washroom.

I smoked hard, and talked with closed lips to the women round me, thinking, I'll be out of here soon, you see? And I won't need her or anyone here. The moment I walk past that gate I'm through, you understand?

When I came out to the Day Room again it was almost empty. The outside door was open. A student nurse sat there, picking at her fingernails.

'Can I go out?'

'Sure. What's your name?'

I told her and she checked my name in the roll book. Then she yelled, 'Miss Willems, here's another one wants to come out.'

Doggie. She makes me sound like a little doggie scratching to go out and lift its leg by a tree.

I tramped down the steps and chose a seat at the far end of the curve of benches. The woman next to me gave me a nudge in the ribs.

'What the hell——?'

She waggled her finger past the row of heads. I saw Miss Willems beckoning to me. I strolled over.

'Yes?' My voice was cool.

'I've been looking for you.' Her face had an impish smile. Her black eyes twinkled. (*Good. She missed me. Serves her right.*) You're going home tomorrow.'

'What?'

You heard it you heard it but make her say it again.

'I said you're going home tomorrow. I saw the memo when I came on duty.'

All the hate went out of me. I sat down heavily.

'I've been waiting. Since yesterday. Every minute I've been waiting.'

'Were you worried?'

'Not worried. Just anxious.'

'You didn't have to be. We all knew you'd pass.' She squeezed my hand.

If I had only waited in the Day Room, she would have told me then. All that stupid anger for nothing. So sweet this is. So right. That she should be the one to bring the news. Look at her. She's happy for me. Really happy.

'Thanks, Miss Willems. Thanks. What time tomorrow, do you know?'

'No, honey. I don't.'

'Did they call my husband on the telephone?'

'I don't think so. They usually send a letter from the Superintendent's office.'

'Would he get it so soon?'

'Now stop your worrying. He'll be here. I'm going to miss you, Judith.'

'Oh, so you want me to stay, is that it?' I quipped, to hold off a choking throat.

She laughed. 'Of course not. I mean I like you. I liked you right off——'

'When I tried to kill myself?' I dropped my eyes.

She touched my hand again. 'Now don't think about that. It's over. You're going home. Everything's going to be all right.'

'Do you know you were the only one who cared?'

'We all cared, honey. We did.'

'But you showed it.' My eyes were still looking down. 'I want to thank you for everything.'

'Just you stay well.' She patted my hand.

'I'll try.'

Tell me move a mountain and I'll try. Tell me walk on my head and I'll try. I love you. Like a mother I love you. I've got a mother but I love you.

She studied her watch for a long moment. Did she sense how I felt?

'Oh. Three-thirty already.' Then she sang out, 'Ward A

girls! Time to wash for cafeteria. Let's go. We'll be out again tomorrow.' She stood up and gathered her charges together. I trailed behind her, watching the sunshine glint on her glossy hair.

I love this woman. She gave me kindness. I will never forget her.

Tonight will be the last time I sleep in a room with thirty others. The last time my sleep will be broken by a scream or a sob of anguish. The only crying I will hear will be that of Gary hungry for food. The only anguish will be my own.

Jay knows it. I'm not well. Merely over the hump of acute depression. Out of the valley of the shadow. When he takes me home tomorrow I will be as I was on my week-end passes, as I was in those first few weeks after the baby was born. I'll ask a million questions. I'll plunge into every task with a flurry and a fury. I won't rest until every loose thread is pulled into place and I am in control again. I won't take it easy. I can't take it easy. I don't know how.

I feel like a racehorse champing at the bit, waiting for the jockey's jab in the flanks to send him hurtling down the track. My goal is acceptance of my baby. This much I know. But why did I fail? What forces were loosed? How can I prevent their recurrence?

I've walked through the ward tonight, looking at familiar things. The crack in the wall in the small ward where I slept until yesterday. The drawer in the dresser in the utility room. It sticks and squeaks. You have to pull it out just so. The tap that needs an extra turn to send the water out. The table in the Day Room where somebody carved her name in the soft wood. The toilet that doesn't flush well. The cracked mirror in the big ward that give you two mouths and two noses and four eyes. I know every sight and sound and feel of A Ward. If I were struck blind tonight, I could move through this little world with confidence.

I wish, how I wish, I could carry this feeling, this safety, this confidence back home.

Thursday, September 21

They've watched me all morning with those hungry, aching eyes. They said good luck and we'll miss you and think of us,

Judith, and they asked me to write. When Beverly took down my home address she said, 'When I get out, I'll come to see you. All right?'

'Sure, Bev. Sure.' I hope she doesn't.

'I'd love to see your little Gary. I'll be lonely without you.'

'You'll be home soon, Beverly. You're off shock. Maybe next week you'll go to Staff.'

'Maybe. But what will I do without you? You're my only friend.'

Why does she talk like that? I can't look at her. It hurts and annoys me.

'You'll make others. I know you will. Oh, Bev, there's the attendant. She wants me. I'll see you before I go.'

'You promise?'

'I promise.'

Millie was in the corridor sitting on a suitcase.

'Is that mine, Millie?'

'Sure, it's yours. You think I'm gonna let you go with somebody else's bag? Don't you remember it?'

'No. I mean, it's been a long time. I——'

'I'm gonna check off your stuff. Then you can pack it up.'

She unlocked the closet door, hopped on a ledge, and scooped out the contents of my bin.

I watched her as she checked out the clothes against a mimeographed list.

Check-out time. Please leave your keys at the front desk. Guests are reminded that the management assumes no responsibility for lost articles. We thank you for your patronage and trust you will favour us again when next you are in . . .

So many clothes. Barely remember them. And so few of them worn. But they're mine. Each piece is stamped with my name in indelible ink that won't wash out. Nice memento.

'Pict-chur a penthouse . . . a-way in the sky . . . with millions of dum-de-dum—da-da-de-die . . .' She was singing softly. 'O.K. Now. Oh, damn. I forgot the stuff in your cabinet in the ward. Put these in the bag. I'll be right back, y'hear?'

She didn't come right back. She must have been delayed on another errand. And I sat there, thinking how ironic it was, spending part of my last hours here surrounded by clothing and personal possessions, symbols of my terrible phobia. Eight weeks ago I wanted to be naked, to wear nothing, touch nothing. I've worn state clothes all this time, except for visits home and to Staff. Now I can finger my things and feel no fear. But I know this clothes phobia and all the others are merely quiescent. They're waiting for me, waiting for another depressive episode. Wish I were in a doctor's office now, talking my heart out. No. Not my heart. My mind. The heart is just a muscle. All this business of loving with the heart . . . you're breaking my heart . . . crying my heart out. The song-writers perpetrated the hoax of the heart. I did, too. I used to write songs. It's more romantic to associate emotions with a fat, red heart than a dirty grey mass of convoluted brain tissue. And you can't rhyme too well with the word brain. Pain. Insane.

Why doesn't Millie come back? Don't like sitting here alone. Look at all those names . . . Johannson . . . Miguel . . . Zyvorg . . . Bruckner . . . adhesive-tape names. There's Hunter, Josephine. My companion of the night. She set her hair and filed her nails last night, sitting cross-legged on the bed like a lioness preening. And when the nurse put out the light she drew up the covers like an obedient child and closed her eyes. Her adhesive tape is yellow. The letters are smudged. She's been here a long time. Years maybe. A caged half-woman. Why do they keep her here in A Ward—to carry out garbage pails each morning?

'O.K., girl, let's snap it up.' Millie came in with a small cardboard box. She dumped my toilet articles on a stool.

'Millie, would you put them in the bag for me? I need a cigarette.'

'What's the matter? You nervous?'

'A little.'

'O.K. I'll put 'em in and set the bag in the office. You grab a smoke. But if Miss Spence catches you, don't snitch on me, y'hear?'

'I won't. Thanks.'

'Wait a minute. You still luggin' that thing around?' She pointed to my knitting bag.

'Yes. Do you mind?'

'Hell, no. You're just a funny one, that's all. Real funny.' She shooed me out.

'Millie, if my husband comes——'

'Don't worry. We'll find you. You can't go far. This is a locked-up place.'

... I'm sitting on an empty bed at the far end of the main ward. The sun is on this bed and it's very warm. But I'm cold and shivering. That woman in the bathroom. The words she said. Why did I have to walk in there?

I never saw that woman before. She must have come on the ward just this morning. I heard her before I saw her. Her voice was so sharp it cut through the babble like a knife. And I couldn't shut my ears or walk away.

'... I'm an alcoholic. They're going to try Antabuse on me ... have to give it in a hospital, you know—powerful stuff. ... Nah, I'm not afraid. I want to stop. ... Girls, how's the food here? Oh, never mind ... I know I won't each much once they start treatment. ... What? oh, Pittsburgh. Yeah, I live there. Say, any of you know Bertha Mayers? She's here, isn't she? I think it was here at State they sent her. I followed the case in the papers. My brother-in-law is a cop. He was one of them who pinched her ... she kidnapped a baby. ... Yeah, swiped it right off the street ... wheeled it away from in front of a store. ... Well, girls, who knows the ropes here? Any of the beds broken? The plumbing leak? Who's got a cigarette ... I can't mooch hooch here ...'

. They laughed and three women offered her cigarettes.

Evil Evil. Lying gossip. Maybe she knows Bertha and hates her. And made the whole thing up from a drunk-sick mind. I don't believe a word of it. And yet. And yet ... Bertha's still in coma. She won't come out of it for an hour or more. I may be gone by then.

But it could be true. It just could. She cried so much last week. Maybe Doctor Manning rehashed the whole thing and told her she'd have to take insulin shock. If it's true, she's sick. Very sick. That story she told me about her husband. Maybe she's not even married. And that picture of her baby. Did she steal that the way she stole the real baby?

But she taught you to play cards. Encouraged you to talk. Made you laugh. Don't hate her. If she did it, she had a hunger so strong it knew no bounds of reason or restraint. She wanted a baby.

I have a baby. And I have yet to learn to want it.

Sitting in the Day Room now. Mouth hurts from smiling. Tired of nodding 'yes, thanks . . . no, I won't forget you . . . yes, I'm happy . . . sure, I'll write . . . thanks again . . . yes, he'll be here soon . . .'

I'm still in this locked-up place, as Millie called it. In a few hours I'll be home. No locks on the doors or bars on the windows. Still I feel as though I'm exchanging one prison for another. This is my place of punishment. Home is the source of my crime. Gary Edward Kruger. My son. Your mother's coming home, Gary. But she really doesn't want to. She's still afraid. She's coming home because there's nowhere else to go.

10 p.m.

The compulsion to finish this hospital diary forces me to write. My release is not a full or final one. When Jay reported to the Superintendent's office this morning they told him I would be under the supervision of a social worker for one year.

'Will she come to the house?' I asked him.

'No, sweetie. You're supposed to check with her at a local hospital. But they know I'm a doctor and that you'll be under therapy. She'll probably call on the phone a few times. That's all.'

'What happens if I . . . if things don't go well?'

'They will.'

'What happens? I want to know.'

'If you have a relapse within a year they'll readmit you without commitment. But——'

'Oh boy. What a break. They'll keep my bed warm for a whole year.'

'Sweetie, I told you you won't go back. Don't think of it.'

I tried not to. Instead I remembered the final moments. I had just joined the line waiting to go outside before lunch when Mrs. O'Neill walked to the head of the Day Room and motioned to me. I felt the sweat pour down my back. My feet moved across the floor as if I were walking through water. The suitcase was sitting in the corridor.

'Are you ready, Judith? Your husband's coming up in the lift.'

'Yes. Do I wait here?'

'Right here. He has the papers for your release.' Then she reached for my hand and pumped it professionally. 'Good-bye. Good luck. And don't come back.' She smiled in her sudden fleeting way.

'I'll try not to.'

She looked at the clock. 'Well, I have to get ready for the insulin group. They'll be out any minute now.'

'Please give my regards to the nursing staff. You've—they've been . . . nice to me.'

Nice. A mealy word to cover a lie and a truth.

'I will. Oh, there's your husband.' She walked into the office.

Afraid to turn round. Hot with embarrassment. Always like this when we meet. As though I were facing a stranger.

'Hi', he said.

'Hi.'

'All ready?' He reached for the suitcase. 'Everything's here?'

Yes. He is a stranger. Why doesn't he ask me if I'm happy or nervous or tell me how glad he is to be taking me home. Something. Anything.

The doors opened from one of the insulin wards. I saw rumpled beds, yards of restraints heaped on the floor, instrument tables cluttered with bottles and syringes. The nurses were leading out the patients now. They were barefooted. They slipped and weaved, still drugged and stuporous. The corridor began to fill up.

Suddenly I was swamped with fear. They're coming after me, to put me back in a bed and tie me down and all the terror and panic will return.

I touched his arm with trembling fingers. 'Let's go. I'm ready. Let's go.'

'Sure. I was waiting for you.' He rang the lift bell.

Why doesn't it come up? Why can't I hear it? In a minute it'll be too late. In a minute——

I closed my fingers on his wrists. He gave me an everything-will-be-all-right smile. Then the door opened. I moved inside quickly.

Sunlight was streaming through the windows of the empty reception room.

'I thought there would be a nurse at the door, didn't you, Jay?'

'Once you clear with the main office, I guess that's that.'

'What time is it?'

'Ten-forty. Why?'

'I just wanted to know.'

Ten-forty. September 21st. A moment in time. Anybody's time. And mine.

The gravel crunched under our feet. He was silent. I wondered if he was thinking, well, here she is. I'm taking her home. This is my wife. Is she a whole person again?

'Look! There they are.'

'Who?'

'Over there. On the lawn. The patients from my ward.' My throat closed up with a sudden spurt of loyalty. From where we were they looked so tiny, a group of huddled figures sitting on the benches under the big tree. Blobs of yellow, red, and blue flashing bright against the dark of the grass. Specks and flecks. They looked so small and lost and trapped.

'Can I wave to them?'

'Sure. If you want to.'

'Yes. I want to.'

Why did I ask him? Why am I afraid of my behaviour when I'm with him?

I waved my arm and waggled my fingers at the group.

Hey, look. It's me. I'm walking with my husband. He's taking me home. Can you see me, Helen, Beverly, Esther, Florence—all of you out there and inside, too? I won't write to you, girls. I'm sorry. I can't. But I'll remember you. With pity, with pain, aud even with love. We need love. We need time. We need help. God, we need help!

The ground dipped a little and they were out of sight. Two tall stone pillars stood at the end of the road.

'Is this the main entrance?'

'Yes. The car is right over there, beyond the gate.'

'What is this building we're passing?'

'The Administration Building. That's where I went this morning. Here's the car. How do you feel? Happy?'

'Very happy. It's good to go home.' I smiled at him.

He put the suitcase in the back, helped me in, and then

walked round to the driver's side of the car. When he slid behind the wheel I blurted, 'Jay, I . . . I'm not really happy. I'm scared.'

'I know you are, sweetie. But that's all right. It'll subside. Just give it time. I saw Doctor Downey at the hospital yesterday. I told him you were coming home.'

'What did he say?'

'He was glad, of course. And I told him you'll call him for an appointment in a few days.'

I was silent.

'You will, won't you?'

'Oh, yes. Sure.'

I have to. That's how I got out of here. With cross-my-heart promises to start therapy right away.

'What's the matter? Don't you like him? Do you have confidence in him?'

'I hardly know him. I saw him twice in the Philadelphia hospital. Whatever he told me, it didn't help.'

He started the car. 'Therapy really begins when the acute stage is over. It's like a fever. Sometimes you can't stop it from rising. When it breaks that's when you start on medicine to speed up recovery. Psychotherapy is medicine, sweetie.' He turned to me and smiled and then eased the car in to the main stream of traffic.

I watched his face. There was intelligence in it. And strength. 'I wish you were my doctor.'

'Will you call Dr. Downey, Judy?'

'I will. I will. Just give me a few days, huh? Don't push me, please.'

It's almost midnight now. I can hear Gary snuffling from the next room. Wonder if he's catching a cold. Would like to unpack my suitcase and put everything away, but it's too late. Can't sleep. There are no sedatives in the medicine chest. I expected that. Jay said he'd give me one when I really need them. I need them now. Can't wake him up. He needs his rest. He didn't approach me tonight. Just a good-night kiss, cool, dispassionate. He must have sensed I'm not ready. Not the first night home.

My father is here. Was surprised to see him but I shouldn't have been. It's just like him. He took an extra day off to welcome me home. Wish he hadn't done that. He's losing pay. Makes me more beholden. Every gesture, every sacrifice they make grinds me deeper in debt to them. How can I make it up? How can I repay?

It's getting chilly. There's winter in the wind. Don't like winter. Or rain, or snow, or life and living. Everything frightens me.

Wonder who's in my bed tonight? Is it a new one? Do they miss me in the ward? It wasn't so bad there. Except for the shock treatments. They made no demands as long as I followed the rules. Now I have to put out again and produce. Groom myself for taking over all alone. Mother can't stay here indefinitely. I said something at supper about it. She answered, 'You're home five hours. Already you're worried when I go back to the Bronx. There's nothing there for me. I want to be here.'

'But Dad is all alone. He——'

'He's not alone. He eats by Cousin Rose twice a week. Every Thursday he works late in the store and——'

My father broke in. 'Darling, look at me? Do I look undernourished?' He chuckled.

'That's not it, Dad. It's a broken life. I broke it up for you.'

Mother pushed her coffee cup away. 'You didn't break it up. And it's not for ever. Just until you're well.'

'That's it. Don't you see? I'm not well. I don't know when I will be. I'm still sick. I'm still nervous.'

They exchanged sharp glances.

'Mom will stay as long as you need her', my father said. He was pushing breadcrumbs into little piles on the tablecloth.

'You want me, don't you, Judith?' she asked.

'Of course I want you. I need you.'

It's true. You're helpless. If she left now you'd fall apart again in twenty-four hours. So why make it hard for them? Why keep harping on it? To show them how guilty you feel? Think I've been guilty since I've been born. But for what? What have I done?

Can't stop writing. Can't let a day pass unrecorded. Have to chronicle everything or I'll lose the full import of this time, this strange, sick time. Maybe I'm torturing myself needlessly this way. I don't know.

My premonition in the hospital was correct. I'm just as I imagined I would be once I came home. Possessed with the devil of obsession. Must know everything, learn everything, do everything. The clock is a whip. Drives me from one chore to another.

'Take it easy', Jay says. 'Let your mother take care of Gary. Go for a walk. Read a little.'

That's a laugh. They brought me back to the root of my sickness and they want me to relax. Feel as I did right after Gary was born. A shadow away from panic. And the panic came and they took me away and now I'm back and what next? Will the circle come full round again?

My diarrhœa is worse. Eyes burn as if I hadn't slept for days. And I haven't. And now there's something new. Massive sneezing attacks. It's not hay fever. Yet the weeds are high in the back-yard. Like a jungle. When Mother goes out to hang up clothes, she's knee deep in them. Gary's growing, too. Fast. Too fast.

In the hospital I ached for freedom. Now I'm free. But I'm hardly outside. I scurry from room to room. I peek at the world from behind drawn blinds. Some nights, when it is dark and there is no moon, I sit on the back steps and stare at the sky.

Called Doctor Downey two days ago. He sounded pleased to hear from me. Professional voice, of course. Have an appointment for next Monday. Don't want to go, but promised Jay that I would. Anyway, I'm not fully discharged. Merely on parole. Maybe they have ways of checking up.

Jay's on O.B. service now. He's home very little. It's selfish, but I'm glad I don't have to make dinner for him every night. Trying to organize a meal is torture. My hands have started to shake again. I've cut myself twice paring vegetables. I drop things. I spill things. The only thing these hands are good for are wringing and writing.

Friday, September 29

When the doorbell rang, Mother was warming the bottle for Gary's lunch. 'I'll take it', I called out.

Beverly was standing there. Beverly Vaughn. From A Ward. I stared, seeing and not seeing, believing and not wanting to believe.

'Hello, Judy. Surprised?' She was wearing a tan belted trench-coat and a scarf on her head. She looked jaunty and well composed.

'Surprised?' I echoed. 'Oh, yes. Very. (*Go away. I left you in the hospital. You're a ghost. A resurrection. Please go away.*) Come in.'

'Is it all right?' The brightness fled from her eyes and her shoulders sagged a little.

'Sure. It's all right.'

'I'm living with my aunt in Willow Grove. That's pretty near, you know. I came in to Philadelphia today. I just took a chance.'

We walked into the kitchen. 'Mother, I want you to meet Beverly Vaughn. She was with me at the hospital. In the same ward.'

'Hello, Beverly', my mother said. Her eyes showed fear and I knew she was thinking, why did you come here, Beverly? You'll excite her. You'll stir her up and make her nervous. She's nervous enough as it is.

'Sit down, Bev', I said. 'Some coffee, maybe?'

'No, thanks. I can't stay long. Is . . . is Gary here? Could I see him?'

Mother looked wary and uneasy. I made a quick gesture with my hands meaning, what can I do? She's here.

'Yes. He's in the other room. I'll show you.'

She watched him for a long moment. He was kicking his feet frog-like against the side of the bassinet. She touched his fingers.

'You have a beautiful son.'

'I know.'

Want him, Bev? You'd love him, wouldn't you, as much as the baby you had to give to your sister.

Mother came in, with a bottle and nappy. 'Excuse me, Beverly. I have to feed the baby.'

'Let's go in the kitchen', I said. 'You sure you won't have anything?'

'No. Really.' When she sat down at my table, the sense of unreality heightened. I thought, a week ago we were at State together. Now she's in my kitchen.

'When did you get out, Beverly?'

'A few days after you did. They gave me another shock two days before that. I didn't want it. I made a real fuss. I ran up and down the ward. They had to catch me.' She dropped her eyes and smiled sheepishly.

'Really? You shouldn't have. (*Lucky fool. You made a big stink and still they let you go.*) Were you nervous at Staff?'

'Oh, terribly. But I prayed. Like I prayed for you.'

Now ask her. Get real chummy and ask her why she was admitted. The whole story. And talk about Bertha and Esther and Florence. Make her stay for lunch. Or make a date for next week. She wants that. She'd like that.

I crumpled a paper napkin. 'Well, I . . . oh, is that Gary? He's a little fretful today. I better see if my mother needs help. I——'

She stood up and collected her purse and gloves. 'I have to go. I got to register with some employment agencies. You know, I used to work at the City Hospital, right here in Philly. I was a Nurses' Aide. Sort of. I helped on the wards. I didn't like it. The sick people made me cry. Now I'm going to try office work. I hope I get something.'

She had that same beaten look in her eyes that she had in the hospital. I wondered if I looked the same to her.

'It was very nice seeing you, Beverly. Come back again some time when you get the chance.'

'Thank you', she said.

We walked to the door. Suddenly she grabbed my hand. 'You were good to me, Judy. You listened. You didn't laugh. You were my friend. God bless you.'

She closed the door softly. I peered through the blinds and watched her go down the porch steps. She didn't look jaunty any more.

Monday, October 2

First session with Doctor Downey. Thought I had forgotten what he looked like. But when he opened the door it seemed like yesterday and not two and a half months ago that I had talked with him.

'Well, hello! How are you, Judith?'

'All right, thanks.' I gave him a weak smile.

'Come in.'

I sat on the edge of a big leather chair and stuffed my coat behind me. He leaned back in his chair and propped his feet on the desk.

He's so relaxed, it's disgusting.

'You're feeling better?'

'A little. But I'm still scared of the baby. My mother takes care of him.'

'She's still with you?'

'Oh, yes.'

Fool. Did you think I'm on my own? You don't know how sick I am. You didn't know three months ago and you don't know now. It's no damn good, my being here. You can't help me. I'm here because Jay wants it; because I told them in the hospital . . .

'What are you thinking about?'

'Nothing.'

'How old is your baby now? A boy, isn't it?'

'Yes. He's four months. Doctor Downey, can you help me?'

'I think so. Yes.'

'Why am I so afraid? Not only of the baby. I stare at people's gloves and pockets and get scared because I know the material is wearing out. I look at their shoes and their run-down heels. I'm afraid of rain and snow and cold. Why?'

'There's an over-all pattern that's more important, I think. These individual fears are symptoms.'

'Oh, yes.'

'You have a brother, don't you?'

'Yes. He's four years younger. He's an architect in Philadelphia.'

Why the hell does he bring my brother into this?

'Do you remember being jealous of him?'

'No. Not at all. I was too busy playing games downstairs with the other children. I wasn't interested in a new baby. I never hit him or resented him. I hardly gave him a thought.'

Satisfied? What are you driving at? Harold isn't in this thing at all.

'And your mother takes full charge of the baby?'

'Most of the time. Or else she watches me as I handle him.'

'How do you feel about her?'

'Feel?'

'Yes.'

'Fine. I mean . . . if it weren't for her . . . She's nervous about Gary. She's an apprehensive person, you know? Like me. We used to fight. I'd get angry when she worried about little things. And I'd yell. But that's all over. I can't get along without her. Some days I'm depressed. Not as bad as before, but bad. I cry a lot. I don't sleep. I was better in the hospital after shock. But I knew it would be like this. All I think of are dirty clothes and shopping and holes and things running down. I used to be so active. So competent. Everyone praised me. I was strong. I'm no good any more. I'm sick. Please . . .'

I cried in front of him. He sat waiting while I blew my nose and wiped the tears away.

'Please, what's wrong? This terror. Of dust and dirt and——'

'Well, as I said before, the trouble is not so much with the specific fears. There's a pattern we have to work on. Compulsions are symptoms. The roots lie deep. The family situation. (*No use. He doesn't understand. He's skirting, hedging. No use at all.*) Judith, I wanted this first visit to be brief. I know you're still upset. How about the same time next week?'

I stood up. 'Doctor Downey, about the fee. I——'

'Suppose we say five dollars a visit.'

'Thank you. Thanks very much. I appreciate it.'

Smile the ever-overgrateful smile with the quiver in the voice and the thanks-for-the-hand-out look in the eyes. Puppy-dog eyes.

He walked with me to the door. 'Think about the few things we mentioned. And try to handle the baby more. By yourself.'

'Yes. Surely. I know that's important.'

Yeah, teach', sure, teach', anything you say, teach'.

I walked through the streets and I remembered how I was down South bucking the crowds, scurrying from one store to the next with shopping lists. Buying things, returning things, watching the clock. A bus to catch. A meal to cook. Letters to write. Busy, busy. No time for fear. Now I trudged like a horse with blinkers, afraid of people, store windows, cinemas.

There was a school near the corner where I waited for the bus. The children were coming out. I thought, kids. Uniforms, books, clothes. They always need something new. Something I can't handle. They need love and attention and care. It's too much for me. Everything is too much for me. Look at that man. He needs new shoes. He's standing there smoking and doesn't even care. But I do. All the time. And Downey tells me to think about my brother and my mother. The family. Doesn't he know the trouble's right here, with this man and his shoes and clothes and my baby?

When Jay called from the hospital to ask me how it went, all I could say was, 'He's only going to charge five dollars a session. Isn't that nice?'

See, Jay. I'm not such a burden. I'm sick, but cheap-sick. First a state hospital and now a doctor who gives you a break in fees. And a mother-in-law who asks no salary. So don't be angry with me. I hate myself enough for two.

Saturday p.m., October 14

Haven't told anyone. I sit by myself and flush with shame when the feeling crawls over me like a snake in the brain. And it's worse when I hold Gary in my arms and cuddle him. My parents smile. They think I mean it; that I am content; that soon everything will be all right. They don't know I'm trying to squeeze myself into a mould, and how hard I'm trying to play the role of a mother. I don't want this part. *I don't want it.* I'm not made for it, that's all. I want to be free. In the world again. To mix with adults. I want kicks and thrills. From the outside. There's nothing here for me. Housework is drab and demanding and unrewarding, and I hate it. And now it's too late because I have a baby and I don't want a baby and I can't give him back. This is terrible. And evil. Because I am evil. I can't tell this to anyone, even Jay. He'll think he married a misfit and he'll be right.

Doctor Downey still harps on getting to the roots of my problems. I continue to beleaguer him with demands for relief from fear. How does he expect me to sit quietly and talk about my family history when I'm scared all the time?

The last time I was there I pressed my nose against the

window of the waiting-room and stared at the street ten storeys below. The old terror, the big terror gripped me. I wanted to jump out. Yesterday I was organizing the cabinet under the sink and saw a bottle of roach killer. I couldn't tear my eyes from the word 'poison'. I stare at knives and broken bottles and razor blades and ice picks.

And he wants me to analyse and be introspective.

Monday, October 23

Jay called this evening and asked me to meet him in the doctor's library. This was the first time I've been in his hospital. I forgot his directions for reaching the main floor corridors. I made a wrong turn and became lost in the long, hot hallways. Almost in panic, I retraced my steps and came to the Admissions desk. Directly across the aisle was a small sign reading 'Staff Library'.

I thought the room was empty, and then I saw him in a far corner. He was sitting deep in a leather chair, his fingers steepled in front of his face. He looked small and tired.

'Jay?' I spoke in a hushed voice.

'Hi.'

I sat next to him in a straight-backed chair.

'I nearly got lost. Maybe I came in the wrong door.'

'Well, anyway, you're here.'

He sat still, his eyes focused on the tips of his fingers. I grew uneasy.

'I ... er ... I saw Doctor Downey today.'

'Anything new?' He still didn't turn to me.

'No. The same thing. He's not helping me.'

He shifted his body. Now I saw his mouth. It was tight.

'Are you trying to help yourself?'

'W-what do you mean? Of course I am. I'm trying to get well. I go to the doctor the way you want me to. I handle the baby. I help a little. I keep going.'

There's something wrong. He's going to tell me he doesn't love me any more.

He unbuttoned the back of his jacket collar and hunched deeper in the chair.

'I know you're trying. I'm not blaming you. Things are

what they are, that's all. It's going to take more time than I thought. I've been thinking about this summer. About going back South to the University. I think it's out.'

I swam in a mixture of fear and relief. But I spoke the right words first. The words he had a right to expect.

'But your residency there. You'd get an easy acceptance.'

'There are other residencies. Philly is a good training area for internal medicine and . . .'

'But you planned it. It was all set.'

Talk and keep talking. Don't let him see you're happy. Is that it? Happy?

'Yeah. I know I planned it. But when things happen you have to change your plans.'

'It's me, isn't it?'

'Yes. In a way. But I'm not blaming you, you understand. Things change. Circumstances come up. So you alter your plans. It's not your fault.'

'I feel guilty. Terribly guilty. (*You don't. You're lying. For this you have no guilt. You never wanted to go back there, did you? But you didn't have the guts to tell him, to cross him, to make him angry and resentful. And you still can't do it.*) Maybe I'll be well enough. It's not until next June.'

Soothe and smooth him. Let him think you're on his side, just as you always were.

'I'll have to see how things go. But it's a possibility. I just wanted you to know how things stand.' He stood up and buttoned his collar. 'I have to check on a patient in the O.B. ward. Can you get out of here all right?'

'Sure.'

'I'll call you tomorrow. I'm off duty tomorrow night. We can talk some more about it then.'

'O.K. Good night, Jay.' My voice was small and contrite. 'You're not angry with me? For spoiling your plans?'

'Of course not! Now listen, don't feel so guilty. Maybe I shouldn't have told you. The main thing is that you get well. Everything'll work out.'

He is standing over me and he cannot see the joy in my eyes. He is thinking of me and I think only of myself. But I'm not bad, am I? Or selfish? I'm sick. Depression turns you in to yourself. And you're not

really happy. Just relieved of the threat of another change, another move.
Your world is so tight and tormenting. He's loosened a link in the chain.
That's all. You love him and you're sorry and guilty. Feel it. For God's
sake you must feel it!

I saw him glance quickly at the doorway. Then he squeezed
my hand. 'Good night, sweetie. I'll call you.'

I sat straight in the chair. The snakes of evil were crawling
again.

Monday, October 30

When he came off duty he looked excited. His eyes were
bright and he walked with a quick, light step.

'Judy, I'm free from tonight until Monday morning. Let's
go up to New York for the week-end. We can leave tomorrow
and——'

My mother must have heard him from the kitchen. She
rushed in. 'Good! Fine! Go ahead', she said. 'Dad'll be here
tomorrow night. You'll have the apartment to yourselves. Call
your friends. Eat out. It'll be good for you. A change.'

He seemed to glare at her for an instant. Then he went on.
'You don't have to. I just thought you'd like it.'

'All right. O.K. It's a good idea.' I left them there and ran
to the bedroom.

Which dresses which shoes which slips which coats . . . two miles
or two thousand . . . must be organized . . . where I go is not important.
Things are important . . . they must be right . . .

I dragged up a suitcase from the cellar and started a list. It
was eleven o'clock.

'You have tomorrow morning to pack', Jay said. He was in
his pyjamas. I knew he wanted me to come into bed with him,
but I couldn't. I had to do it now. If he tried to stop me I
would have screamed and hit him.

As I scurried from closet to suitcase, I thought, Home. I
haven't been there for a year and a half. What will it look like?
How will I feel?

The car rolled down the bridge ramp from Manhattan to the
Bronx. On Mitchell Avenue now . . . there's Linden Street . . .
now Kelway . . . closer, closer . . . there's the Library on the

corner . . . when I was eight it seemed so big and wonderful . . .
looks small now . . . turning down the block now . . . stomach
turning, too . . . scared . . . why am I scared . . . this is my old
neighbourhood . . . the signs and streets and stores and smells of
yesterday . . . a thousand yesterdays . . . the candy store. Please,
Mr. Rosen, put plenty of sprinkles on my cone, huh? Eyes big
and greedy, watching him twirl the ice-cream in the nest of
chocolate . . . Delicatessen. Ripe, rich odours of nuts and
halvah, smoked fish and salami.

The car turned on to my street . . . two blocks farther . . . now
just one. Slowly now, slowly . . . Jay eased to the kerb and
pulled up the brake and turned to me, smiling. 'Well, you're
back home, sweetie. How do you feel?'

'Fine.' I licked my lips and swallowed the gorge of fear.
When he slammed the car door shut I jumped.

'What's the matter?'

'Nothing. You just shut doors too loud.'

I looked up at the house. White bricks now streaked with
grey. Twenty-eight years old. As old as I am. Mother was
pregnant with me when she walked up the boards over new-laid
cement in the court. My house. I know every brick in it. Funny
how shock didn't blur the memory of this. Wonder if the bushes
still bear tiny flowers in the Spring? Do rain puddles still settle
in the courtyard cracks? I used to jump them and laugh. Are
those new curtains on the big door? There, I see my name. My
real one. The first me. Second one up from the bottom. . . . Two
rings, then wait for the buzzer. . . . Mommy, Mommy, hurry
up, let us in. Time for Uncle Don and Buck Rogers and Just
Plain Bill. . . . No buzzer to answer me now. Door pushes open.
Hinges still creak. . . . Turn to the left . . . up three wide steps.
Jay kissed me here on our third date. Kissed me and pressed me
and told me he liked me very, very, very much. . . . The bank
of mailboxes . . . Always waiting for letters from him, from
anyone. So hungry for mail. . . . Now up. White marble steps,
eight to the landing. . . . Top of the steps now. Turn to the
left. Brown door with gold letters. Apt. 2H. This door and no
other.

I fumbled in my purse for the keys Mother had given me.
First the top lock. Hands are shaking . . . forget how to do this

... never had to open the top ... always someone home ...
won't fit ... no, there it is ... now the bottom ... now ...

'Oh, Jay! I dropped the keys, I can't see where they fell.
Jay, I'm so nervous, I don't know why.'

He picked up the keys. 'Do you want me to open it?'

'No. No. I'll do it. There.' I pushed in on the door and
groped for the light switch on the wall.

Jay walked past me to the living-room and put the suitcase
down in the middle of the floor. 'Why stand there in the hall?'

'I'm coming.' I sat down on the couch and ran my hands over
the soft blue plush. I thought, what's wrong with me? Why does
it hurt? Am I ashamed to come home? Twenty-three years here
and I can't look at it now. I flicked my eyes, from room to
room, from ceiling to floor. No. Not ashamed. It's no different
than before. Just needs painting and new rugs. She couldn't get
to it. She's been with me for four months. It's not the place. It's
me. I'm different.

'Jay, I don't feel so good.'

'Why?' He reached for my hand, but I made a fist and
pressed it to my mouth. He pulled it down.

'I don't know. I don't know anything. I'm sick.' I was
standing up now and yelling in his face. 'Sick. Sick. All over
again. Just like before. No good at all. Do you hear me. Do
you?' My voice screamed back at me from the walls. 'I said
I'm SI-I-ICK!'

He caught my hands as I was beating them against my chest.

She keeps asking him what happened, what happened in
New York that made me so upset. And she blames herself for
urging me to make the trip. She had nothing to do with it. ...
He gave me a sedative and made me lie down and rest. Then
I insisted on calling two of my friends. They came with their
husbands that evening. I was quiet now. Too quiet. I sat and
watched them and I smiled when I wanted to cry.

'Nervous', I told them. 'I've been sort of nervous since the
baby was born. My mother is staying with me for a while.' And
then, for an instant, I was tempted to tell them I had tried to
kill myself and had been in a mental hospital. They would raise
their eyes in surprise and sympathy. They would cluck their

tongues. The giggling would stop. The conversation would be forced. And then, after I had left, they would call people on the phone to pass the news along.

'Did you say anything, Judy?' Mother asked. Her eyes were narrow. 'About the hospital and . . . and everything?'

'What do you think? Don't you think I have some sense? Why don't you trust me? What am I, a child?'

'Wait a minute. All I said was——'

'All you said, all you said. You're always accusing me.'

Jay flashed her a sign with his eyes. She turned back to the stove. She's afraid of him. She listens to him as if he were God.

The visit home triggered another chain of fear. For the past four days I've been cowering in bed like a scared rabbit. I tried to make supper for Jay last night. It took me three hours. *Three hours!*

I asked the doctor what happened. But I'm so damn nervous I hardly listen to him when he talks. I think he said something about associations with the past. A stirring up. Then he counters my questions with more of his own, and I'm too upset to think straight.

Each time I come home from a visit with him Mother waits at the door for me, her eyes so big with hope. It hurts and annoys. She's rushing me. Everybody's rushing me. Except Jay. He must know for sure now that I can't go back South next summer.

November 25

When Shirley walked in the years fell away. I saw her and myself as we were at fourteen, scuffing saddle shoes along the streets of the Bronx, arms linked, voices low and giggly, the world and all its people a constant source of fuel for the fires of adolescent ridicule.

We were the voyeurs, the observers and the judges, smug and wise, throbbing with delight as we chewed each morsel of gossip.

I looked at Shirley now. She was still fair and blonde. Her face was fuller, suffused with the glow of girl-turned-woman. In the past six months we had both given birth to our first babies.

I squealed with forced delight. 'Shirley! Hel-lo!'

'Judy!' She giggled. 'How are you? You look wonderful!' Lips brushing cheeks. Hand clutched.

'Come in . . . come in . . .' . . . 'how was the trip?' . . . 'where's the baby?' . . . 'where's yours?' . . . Laughter. Bundles dropping. My mother kissed her and so did Jay. Then Al, her husband, came up the steps, carrying their baby.

'Oh, Shirley, he's precious. Blond, like you.'

She hefted the baby from him and rumpled his hair. 'Look. Curly. Isn't it marvellous? You know my straight hair. Where's Gary?'

'In the back. He's sleeping.'

My father came in and hugged her and she giggled some more and the room rang with the sound of our voices. When she wasn't looking at me, I stared at her.

This is my best friend. We've known each other for fourteen years. Millions of words. Hundreds of letters. Now I hate her. Jealous of her health, her happiness, her adjustment to motherhood. Don't want her here. Don't want any of them. When she called last week I should have made up an excuse. Why do I torture myself like this?

Each time I went to the kitchen to stir a pot Mother trotted after me to ask if she could help. I knew she was watching me, afraid I'd break up, or cry, or run into the bathroom to hide.

And whenever Shirley asked me a question Mother's eyes were sharp and fearful. She didn't have to worry like that. She doesn't know what a good actress I am when I have to be. They never saw me in the hospital, yes-ing and no-ing my way out on good behaviour.

But it was hard. Very hard. As the day wore on the muscles in my chest and neck were coiled like bands of steel.

'Do I remember who? Oh, Mildred? She went to college with you, didn't she? . . . What? Four children? How nice . . . No. I haven't heard from Janice. You know how you lose touch.'

The game of remember who, remember when. We played it all afternoon. We laughed and clucked and took pictures of the babies. We fed them and ate in shifts. And then it was all over. We all trooped out on to the porch to say good-bye. I held Gary in my arms and waved to them as they got into their car.

The little play had ended. I had fooled her completely. Of course I was lucky, too. She hadn't called during the months I was at State. But I could fool the others, too, if I had to—the other friends, the relatives, Jay's family. It's easy to lie when nothing shows on the outside.

November 26

My baby is almost six months old. His skin is pink satin. His hair is like duck down, blowy and soft. His body is warm with the pulse of young life. All this I see and feel. Yet I can give nothing in return. I cannot love with a mother's love. Where there should be love there is hate. Not for him. For myself. For the inability to love. A circle without an end.

November 29

The circle is smaller now. Tighter, blacker, more painful.

Want to kill myself again.

The love and support of Jay and my parents is not enough. Nothing is enough.

I force myself to keep the appointments with Doctor Downey. Am just as miserable after I see him as before. It's not his fault. Or maybe it is. He's the doctor. Why doesn't he help me?

When Jay is home I don't let him sleep. I thrash in my bed and drench it with the sweat of fear. I can't concentrate on anything except the words I write here. And it's hard to hold a pencil. My knuckles are black and swollen. I beat on walls and doors. My head throbs with the blows of my fists. Want to hurt myself. More and MORE and MORE.

December 9

This afternoon I talked to Jay in the hospital library. I sat with him as I would with a stranger. There is nothing left of our original relationship. We've had intercourse once since I came home from the hospital. We don't take walks or go out together. He walks tight-lipped through the house and eats in silence the meals Mother cooks for him. There is no talk of friends, of his internship, of his plans for the future. Since he

decided not to apply for the residency down South he hasn't
spoken of himself or his work.

But he listens to me. He has patience. Patience for the patient.
His first brush with someone who is mentally ill.

'Do you think I'm selfish, Jay? That's all I can think of.
That I'm selfish and no good. That——'

'Hospital property.' He pointed to the medical journal I was
twisting in my hands.

'Oh. Yes.' I smoothed it and put it back on the table. 'Every
day I say it, like a prayer. This is a good, a wonderful thing, to
learn to love your baby. There is nothing more important than
caring for your own. You should be happy. You will be happy.
But it's no good, Jay. Why?'

'Because the brain can't tell the emotions how to feel and
what to do.'

'But I've got to do something! I can't go on this way.'

'It'll get better. I told you before and I still mean it.'

*I know you do. But it's different now. There's no light in your eyes.
You don't hold my hand. You don't smile. The only thing you have
for me is tolerance, a kind of professional tolerance. Still, it is easier to
talk to you than to Mother. She still doesn't understand what happened
to me. But it's not her fault. All the girls she knew, all my friends,
grew up, got married, and had babies. No suicides, no breakdowns, no
shock treatments. And I am the daughter of whom she was so proud.
Talented. Capable. On her own for five years. Everything I did and
was seemed to point towards success as a mother. How can I blame her?*

'You didn't answer me. Am I selfish?'

'I don't know.'

'I must be. There's something wrong with a woman who
can't love her own baby.'

'Maybe fear is covering up your real emotions. The responsibility of someone to care for.'

'Doctor Downey said that last week. And I think he said it the
week before. . . . But it's more than that. I'm not afraid because
he's tiny and helpless. There's something inside of me that's
evil and corrupt. I can't put the baby's needs above my own.
I can't give. I'm locked up. Nothing comes out but . . . but . . .
this.' I held up my trembling hands.

Now he looked at me. 'I know what you're going through. I

really do. It's damn hard to face ourselves and find out what we're like inside. That goes for everybody. Me too.'

'You? You're all right. You're strong. You're not afraid to live. Or love.'

Ask him now . . . now . . . does he love you? Still love you? Ask him.

'Judy, I told you before. We all have our breaking points. I'm not immune to a breakdown. No one is. Now it's happened to you. But you've got to keep trying to understand.'

'Do you want me to?' Tears clouded my eyes.

'Yes. I want you to get well. More than anything I want you well.'

January 4

Now I know why I am sick. He told me to keep trying to root out the truth and I did. I did it huddled in a corner or crying on the bed. I did it beating on the walls, washing nappies, scrubbing down the tub, scribbling a shopping list. I did it in the frenzied moments and the quiet ones.

And now it's out. Slowly, painfully, I've squeezed out truth like toothpaste from a tube. I'm small and flat and empty, yet curiously relieved. I know what I'm going to do.

Jay is far less upset than my mother. When I told them this evening she sat like someone stricken or beaten. All she could say was, 'What happened to the love you both had? What happened? It was there, wasn't it? Wasn't it? So what happened? It doesn't disappear. So what happened?' Over and over. Like a gramophone record with a crack in it.

And every time Jay said, 'I understand', she stared at him as though he were a partner to my crime against myself.

Is it a crime to want to be free? I don't know how to love and take care of those who need me. The feeling I have for Gary is purely sensual. I have no maternal instincts because I am not really a woman. I want to be a breadwinner, and only for myself. Everyone has tried to make me into something I am not fitted for. This kind of acting I cannot do. I'm a misfit in marriage. The only reason I didn't break before was that we had no children. Now we have a child. Jay can't throw the baby out just because I'm incapable of love.

I want to separate, leave him and the baby. Go back home and exist in the only way I can survive. A room in their apartment. A simple job. Responsible for no one other than myself. A small and undemanding life.

Mother can't see it, not in the slightest degree. She babbles of love and being together and throwing my life away and you don't know what you're saying and you won't be happy. I know it. I don't want happiness. I want relief.

When I asked Jay if he were shocked, he said, 'No. I understand how emotional turmoil could make you withdraw.'

He understands. He's smart. But still I wish he *were* upset like my mother, that he'd beg me not to leave, tell me that he needs me, that he won't let me go. Then I could hold his hand and tell him I have to go. He said he wanted me to get well. Is that all? Doesn't he love me?

January 8

'Could you speak up a little, Judith? I can't hear you.'

I coughed, and choked back the tears. 'I said I want to sink. Be bad. Do bad things.' My hands were hanging down between my knees, shredding wet tissues and wadding them in little balls.

'Go on.'

'It's hard to say it.'

'What do you mean, bad things?'

'I told you. I want to leave the baby and Jay and go off by myself.'

'Yes. I know. (*So you know. That's nice. That all you can say? You're just like Jay and all the doctors. Sounding boards. Echo chambers. Human wailing walls.*) Do you want to go on?'

'I know what will happen to me.' My voice droned in a monotone. 'I'll become evil. Turn into a prostitute. Lie in the gutter and be dirty.'

'Judith, I'm sorry. I still can't hear you.'

'The gutter! I said I want to lie in the gutter.'

Hear me now? What should I do? Shout from the roof that I'm filthy and evil?

'I see. (*O.K. Write it down in my folder. 'Patient wants to prostitute self.' Very pretty, huh?*) Why do you feel this way?'

'I just do.' The tears were there again, rolling down my cheeks. I took off my glasses and ground the soggy tissues into my eyes.

'Do you think you're trying to punish yourself?'

'What?'

'This feeling of moral degeneration . . . the desire for evil . . . it seems to be a form of self-punishment, doesn't it?'

He leaned back. I stared at the ribbing on his socks and the punchwork on the toe of his shoes. I couldn't lift my eyes to him.

'Maybe. I don't know', I mumbled.

'Did you feel this way before your decision?'

'What decision?'

'To leave home.'

So it's final for you, too? You accept it as easily as Jay does. Why don't you try to talk me out of it?

'No, I don't think so', I shrugged. 'Or maybe I did. Everything seemed to come to a head this past week. All the bits and pieces fell together. I saw what I am and what I'm not and that I'm no good for marriage or motherhood.'

'And you think that's evil?'

'Yes.'

'There are many other people who don't fit into a situation in the way it's expected of them.'

'I don't care about other people. I care about myself and what's happening to me.' I looked at my watch. 'I think the time is up.'

He checked the clock on his desk. 'Yes, it is.'

When we stood by the door he said, 'Will you think about what we've discussed?' He touched his hand to my shoulder and I shivered.

'I will. I always do.'

What the hell do you think I do all day?

No use, no use, no use. The lift cables twanged in echo. He can't help me. Or I won't let him. I'm too sick to be helped. The cold winter air whipped my face.

He, too, is willing, I thought. Ready and willing to let me throw my life away. Mother said that, didn't she? And I shouted her down. Maybe she's right. I'll hole up in a corner

and think I'm free. A drawing back. A running away. Like the
sleeping pills and the pieces of glass. But will it be far enough?
Will it bring peace, or more guilt, more hate, more pain?
I've had enough pain. I couldn't stand any more. And I'd
have to pack and travel home, alone. She loves me, but would
she leave the baby and Jay? Jay. How easily I've pushed him
aside and swept everything away in my hunger for relief. Of
course I'm selfish. But sick-selfish. Strangling in the web of
self. If I could open up, break free the right way. If. A thousand
ifs . . . a million hows . . .

January 9

'Hello. Doctor Downey?'

'Yes?'

'Judith Kruger. I——'

'Hello. How are you?'

'O.K. I mean, well, I'm calling to ask you something. Are
you busy?'

'No. Go ahead.'

'You're sure I'm not interrupting anything?'

'No. It's all right.'

'I was wondering . . . after yesterday. I'm all confused.'

'About what?'

'The treatment. I don't think I'm getting better. I mean . . .
(*oh, God, the time you spent planning this and now you fumble!*) . . .
all the things I told you yesterday. Well, I don't want to do
anything hasty. I want to try and work something out. But I
seem to be stalemated. (*Good. That word you remembered.*) I was
wondering if . . . do you think you could recommend another
doctor . . . for an opinion . . . or a consultation?'

*Now he'll have to hate me. My nerve. My gall. My lack of confidence
in him. He's so quiet. Didn't answer. Did he hang up?*

'Yes. If you want to. It's all right with me.'

'Oh, thank y——'

'There's a doctor . . . a colleague of mine. Let me contact
him this evening. I'll try to make an appointment for you.'

'Thank you, Doctor Downey. Should I call you?'

'No. I'll call you tonight.'

'I do appreciate it. Very much. You're not angry?'

'No. Why should I be?'

'Sure.' I tried to laugh. It came out as a grunt. 'You're right. Thanks again. Good-bye.'

January 12

Dr. Lowett's office was in a big building in down-town Philadelphia. As I stepped into the lift I opened my purse to touch the folded sheet of paper inside.

I had typed it the night Doctor Downey called to give me this appointment. It took me two hours to organize the notes from this diary. But now I was so glad I've written things down. It's always good to keep a record . . . you never know when you'll need it.

They saw me typing and asked what I was doing. I told them. Mother was confused. I knew she'd be. But Jay looked sort of pleased.

'I'm glad you're trying', he said.

'Why? I thought you didn't care if I left.'

'I never said that.'

'Yes, you did. In the kitchen that night. You said, you understand and you don't care.'

'I do. I don't want you to leave. But I can't hold you by force. If you think that's the only way you'll get well, I can't stop you.'

I didn't tell him I wasn't going to do it, at least not now. . . .

The door to his waiting-room was open. The room was large and well furnished. I sat down on a modern armless chair with a sharply slanting back. It was very uncomfortable. In a few minutes the inner door opened. Doctor Lowett was a short, fat man in a brown gaberdine suit. The frames of his glasses cut into the fleshy part of his temples and sat deep in the fat of his cheeks.

'Mrs. Kruger?'

'Yes.'

'Come in.' His voice was nasal.

When he motioned me to sit down I was so tense that my vision was constricted. I saw only the outlines of his office. But I felt a thick rug under my feet, and when he sat behind the desk he seemed so far away, across a sea of blond oak.

He picked up a folder, glanced at it briefly, and then leaned back in the chair. Not too far. And he didn't put his feet on the desk. The second before he spoke seemed an eternity. I thought, no hello? No how are you feeling today? No smile? Does he hate me already?

'Doctor Downey sent me a résumé of your case.'

'Yes. But I also brought an outline. I typed it. All the important things. I don't know whether he has them there.' The paper crackled as I unfolded it and handed it to him.

'Why exactly did you want to see me?'

Doesn't he know? Didn't Downey tell him I wanted another doctor's opinion?

'I . . . well, I haven't been getting any better. And I want to leave my husband and baby. Not really. I mean that's how I feel. I can't seem to take hold.'

He scanned the sheet. 'Your husband is a doctor?'

'An intern. Here in Philly.'

He glanced at the paper again. 'And your mother is with you?'

'Yes. Since the baby came. If it wasn't for her I don't know what I would have done.'

'These touching compulsions as a child . . .'

'Eight. I was eight. But they stopped when I went to camp.'

'They are quite common. Expressions of resentment against authority.'

'Who? What authority?' I grew flustered.

'The one the child fears, or hates, or both.' He spoke like a stockbroker reading quotations from a tape.

I thought, how brusque he is, how bored he seems. But he answered my question. I need answers. I hunched forward in the chair.

'What about the phobias, Doctor Lowett? They all came out in the depression. I'm afraid of everything. Cold . . . rain . . . shoes . . . clothes——'

He waved me silent with a small, pink hand. 'They all tie in with the compulsions. The birth trauma broke down the defences.' He stared at me blandly.

Questions massed and bounced off each other. But I couldn't

bring them to expression. Instead I said, 'Defences? Against w-what?'

'Anxiety.'

A mechanical answer man. Push a button and you get the answer. But only for that specific question. No elaboration. If you want to know more you have to push another button. Maybe it's me. I used to learn so well, so fast. Grasped things so easily. But now I'm sick and thick and it's hard to understand what these doctors tell me. He said anxiety. That means nervousness, doesn't it?

'Doctor, why am I afraid of my baby? Why do I want to run away from him and Jay and everything?'

'Because you think you won't be as good a mother as your own mother was.' He pressed the bridge of his glasses with a fat finger.

'Why? What has my mother got to do with it? She's not afraid.'

Just like Downey now. Dragging in the family.

He swallowed a yawn. 'I've seen it many times in other cases. This rivalry between mother and daughter regarding a new baby.'

What is he talking about? She's not jealous of Gary. She wants to help. Why can't I understand him?

My head began to throb in confusion. I kept shaking it as I spoke. 'I've always wanted to give them pleasure. And now I'm not. I always worried about their growing old and dying and——'

'This is an anticipated death wish. It was intensified by the baby.' His voice droned nasally.

Waitwaitwait please. Death wish? What death wish? You're wrong. I don't want them dead. I love them. I need them. Omygod, he's getting up. He's walking to the door. Quick, your purse . . . follow him.

When I got to the door he gave the paper back to me.

'You have to realize your resentment and all your feelings towards them.'

'Doctor, just one more question. Should I continue therapy? I'm not making headway. I see Doctor Downey twice a week now. My husband said maybe more?'

'Doctor Downey is a competent man. You should definitely continue.' He opened the door.

'But——'

'I'll send him my evaluation.' He nodded to a woman in the waiting-room. 'Good-bye, Mrs. Kruger.' His mouth creased in a half-smile and he touched my arm.

'Good-bye, Doctor Lowett.' I stepped aside to let the woman pass. When the door closed on them I heard nothing. It must have been sound-proofed. I stood in the waiting-room for a few moments giving full rein to the pounding in my head. Then I looked at my watch.

Just ten minutes. That's all he gave me. That and the bum's rush. And he was so smug and bored and so damn cocksure.

My steps echoed in the empty hall. I stabbed at the lift button.

All those things he said. About Mother. Showing her up . . . wanting them dead. He's crazy!

January 15

So awkward to see Downey again. Feel like a traitor skulking home. Can't tell him I didn't like Lowett. They are probably friends.

'Well, Judith, how've you been?' Doctor Downey smiled at me. I tried to detect a note of resentment in his voice. There was none.

'The same. I saw Doctor Lowett.'

'Yes. I know. He sent me his report.'

'There were things . . . points he made. I didn't under-stand.'

'What things?'

'About my parents. That my mother is my rival. That I'm competing with her for the baby. That I resent her and my father.'

Thought about it for three days and it's still silly.

He nodded. I said, 'Is it true?'

'I think so. In broad terms, yes. You've told me how you felt about them. This pitying love. There's an element of contempt in there.'

So he's on that too, is he? They're both wrong!

'I don't see what that has to do with not sleeping and why I'm always afraid.'

'You seem to refuse——'

'I *don't* hate them. I hate myself. For being sick and not taking care of the baby and making my mother live with me and leaving my father alone in New York and——'

'You're very much concerned about them, aren't you?'

'Yes. (*And don't you tell me that's wrong because it's not.*) Doctor Downey, am I right in wanting to chuck up everything? My mother tells me I should keep trying. I do try, really. And nothing changes. I lie in bed at night and shake. I'm so knotted inside I——'

'Judith, you're mentally competent. But I don't know if it's right, as you put it. It depends on where you live. You told me there was always tension in your home life. This situation is sure to——'

'Should I get a job?' I cut him off so abruptly I had to apologize. 'They're telling me to get out, to get back to what I say I can do. Handle things in the outside world.'

'It's up to you. If that's what you want.'

How neatly he parries. Throws the hot potato back in my lap. Damn these doctors!

'It's not what I *want*. I want everyone to leave me alone. But if it'll help, I'll try it. I'm not afraid of a job.'

'You'll be going back South this summer, won't you?'

'No. I mean, it's not definite. I didn't tell you. Jay says he may pass up that residency.'

'Why?'

'Because of me. I couldn't take the change.'

'I see. Well, it's still not definite. If you feel you want to try a job for these months, I see no reason why not.'

I can't remember the rest of the session. I sat there, stewing in indecision and hating him for being so vague, and thought, why the hell can't he give me a yes or a no, a word of direction. Show disapproval or support. Something I could hold.

No use no help no good. The grandfather clock in the waiting-room ticked out a pattern of futility.

January 16

'Jay, will you look at me for a minute?'

Reading, always reading. So cool to me, so distant. Even the nights when Mother goes out for a walk. What does he want? I should wake one morning whole and new again?

He closed his book, keeping a finger between the pages.

'I'm not getting anywhere with Downey. Can't I get another doctor?'

'Even after the consultation with Lowett?'

'Yes. I told you.'

'Not much.'

'You didn't ask. You weren't interested.'

'I'm not like your parents. I can't hover and hang over you.'

'It's not that. It's more than that. Everything's fallen apart for us.'

'No, it hasn't.'

'Are you kidding?'

'We're still together. We have an apartment and furniture——'

'You bought it. You did everything.'

'I'm more than six months through my internship.'

'If it wasn't for my mother——'

'But you still want to get out, don't you?'

'Yes. I'm a misfit. The more I try, the worse I feel. I'll never make it. It's seven months already.'

'That's not long.'

'Not for you. You're well. I'm not.'

'Then why do you want to try another doctor? First you tell me you——'

'I know, I know, I know. So it's not logical. So what? I just feel like it. I want another doctor.' I spoke loudly, defiantly, trying to blot out my own confusion.

'O.K. I'll ask around.' He opened the book again.

Time's up. Interview over. Ears shut. Eyes away. Thank you, my husband, for giving me five minutes. If you knew how hard it is to come to you, to ask for things. If only you knew——

Thursday, January 25

'It's raining, Judith.'

'I've got eyes.'

'I mean, you don't have to go today.'

'Look, Mother, you told me to get a job, didn't you?'

'Yes, but why go in the rain?' She was holding Gary in her arms. He was trying to pull out the combs in her hair.

'If I keep putting it off——'

'But today it's——'

'Raining. You said that. Twice already. (*What is it about her? Or me. She rubs me wrong. I yell at her when I want to talk nicely. I pick on every word she says. Why am I so rotten?*) If I keep putting it off, I'll never get out. Here. See? I clipped out five leads from the paper last night.'

'Writing jobs?'

'Why do you say that?'

'Well, that's your line, isn't it?'

'I don't have a line. So I was an editor of a company newspaper. You think I could handle something like that now? What do you want from me?'

'Nothing. I just thought——'

' "You just thought." Here. This is what I'm gong after.' I waved the clippings in her face. 'Sales help. Clerk. General office work. See?'

'Yes. I see.' She pried two combs from Gary's hands and hiked him high on her shoulder.

Now she's angry. I've made her angry. Shouldn't have done that. Scared when she looks like that, when she won't answer.

'Well, I'm going now.' I slipped the umbrella catch and opened the door to the hallway. She took a quick step backward.

'What's the matter?'

'Isn't there a draught?' She was shielding Gary's head with her hand.

Hover, hover, watch and hover. Remember when Harold or I would catch cold? You didn't listen when we talked. You watched our mouths and noses as if they were disembodied things, spreading death in droplets. And if we approached each other you started with those warning signals. A sharp nod, a stepping back, a quick hand to the mouth. If Harold caught my cold you went tsk-tsking all over the house. What did you want me to do, stop breathing?

'I'll be back. Late.' I slammed the door louder than I meant to. And I heard it slam again and again as I sat in the bus, each time with a flicker of fear.

'Hi', Jay said.

'Hello.' I was pinning a dress shield in the armhole of a dress and didn't look up. I talked to myself. (*Brown shoes brush them. Brown pocketbook and gloves . . . check stockings for runs . . . get suspender belt and clean slip . . . necklace and earrings . . . what goes with brown . . . the gold set or——*) 'What? I didn't hear.'

'I said how did it go?'

'O.K. I've got a job.'

'Fine! I'm glad to hear it.'

'A job?' My mother rushed in from the kitchen.

'Yes. Selling for a hotel.'

'You sell the hotel?' she asked. Jay and I laughed.

'No, Mother. I work in the Banquet Department. I run down leads and call up people. Try to get them to book their functions in the hotel. Conventions, sales meetings, office parties. Things like that.'

The voice of Mrs. Meredith, cool and metallic, was still in my ears.

'Who is taking care of your baby, Mrs. Kruger?' Blood-red nails tapping a pencil.

'My mother. She lives with us.'

'I see. And you'll be staying in Philadelphia?'

'Yes. My husband's an intern. Then he'll be in training for internal medicine.'

'How interesting.' She shifted her tightly girdled body in the seat. 'Well, your qualifications seem adequate. It's important that you've had experience in meeting the public.' She made the word public sound indecent; almost dirty. 'Of course you'll be doing most of your work over the telephone. When the leads come in you'll turn them over to me or one of the other women. We take care of all the booking details. We pay one dollar an hour plus 5 per cent commission. After the affair is over. There are cancellations, you know. We don't pay on business which doesn't materialize.'

'Yes. I understand.'

That suit must have cost at least a hundred. And her feet in those shoes. Ankles so slim. Why can't I wear heels like that?

'Most of your phone calls will be in the morning and early

afternoon. Since you preferred part-time work this should work out well.'

'Do you furnish the leads?'

'Most of them. Of course it's up to you to keep your eyes open. Newspapers. The society page. Word of mouth. Friends of yours getting married——' She laughed. It came out through her nose in a sniff. 'That's right. You haven't been here long enough for that. Well, we'll see how it goes. This work is quite interesting. And the commissions should be a nice incentive for you. When do you want to start? Our last solicitor left to join her husband overseas. She only gave me a week's notice.' A corner of her mouth twisted in remembered annoyance.

'Tomorrow?'

'That's Friday. We usually like our help to start on a Monday. But you can come in and help me get her lead cards together. She wasn't very neat. At nine then?'

'Yes.'

A bellhop came in and looked around. He had a sheaf of papers in his hand.

'Here. I'll take that', she said. I saw that they were printed menus. I turned to say good-bye, but she had sat down at the desk again, tapping the papers with her pencil, one eyebrow lifted in disapproval.

'It sounds good', Jay said.

'Just what you wanted', Mother said. Her face was still animated but I saw her hesitation behind her smile. She was waiting for me to reassure her that yes, oh, definitely, it's just what I wanted.

I was excited inside, but I didn't want to show them. Especially her. She gets so involved in everything I do, the shame is twice as bad if something goes wrong.

In bed last night Jay lay with his hands folded under his head, his eyes staring at the ceiling. I looked at his profile. The hate drained out and I shivered with a spasm of desire. When we had been close I would rest my head in the crook of his arm. And then I'd run my hand across his chest and feel the wire roughness of his hair. Then down the body and the leg and up again. A little harder this time. I would press against him, my hands insisting, demanding. Then he'd turn to me. He'd kiss me between my breasts and——

'I spoke to a few people at the hospital today. The pathologist gave me the names of two doctors.'

'Oh?'

'He said they're both good men.'

I shivered again, this time with apprehension. The unknown again. The challenge of decision. I pressed my face into the pillow. Then I asked him, 'What are their names?'

'One is a Doctor Walsh. The other is Doctor Borman. Say, what's the name of that hotel where you'll be working?'

'The Winston.'

He flicked on the bed light, got out of bed, and took his wallet from the pocket of his uniform. Then he flipped through a small notebook.

'Here it is', he said.—'Walsh is at North 39th. Borman is nearer the centre of town. Closer to your hotel.'

Settled. Borman it is. Like picking names from a hat. Chance and circumstance.

He ripped out the page. 'I'll leave this here for you.'

'Yes. That'll be fine.'

Fine and dandy, sugar candy. Whoops! Off to the races. Rat races. Round and round she goes and where she stops . . . ?

He switched off the light and got back into bed. 'You'll call Borman tomorrow?'

'Yes. Tomorrow.'

'G'night. Try to get some sleep', he said.

'Jay?'

'Mmm-n.'

'I've been thinking. Maybe there's no private phone at work. I don't know the set-up there. Could you call Borman for me? Please? Make an appointment for any afternoon.'

'O.K. I'll try to call.'

'Thank you.'

'It's all right. G'night. Get some sleep.'

Get some. Wait on the corner of consciousness. Then reach out and grab sleep. No. Play it cagey. Make believe you don't care if it never comes because you have nothing to do tomorrow. Make your mind a blank, a zero. Lie so still sleep won't know you're waiting.

At one-thirty I had to ask Jay for two sleeping pills.

Friday, January 26

'The job's all right, Mother, but I don't like her.'

'Who?'

'My boss. Mrs. Meredith. She's snooty and cold. A stick. Like a frozen stick.'

I saw those bloody nails again, plucking cards from my hands as I went over the file of leads, and her eyes, slitted and waiting, as she watched me make my first telephone call. And her heels clicking when she walked to me, and her voice, as she spoke with controlled sharpness. 'Here we don't ask them if they've made arrangements yet. You make it so easy for them to say yes, the way that one did.' She pointed to the telephone. 'Tell them we're holding so-and-so date open and we'd like them to come in and make final arrangements. And you don't have to give them your name. Just say Winston Hotel. Do you understand?' She flipped the card over. 'Now try another one.' ...

'You'll stay, won't you?' Mother said.

'Yeah, sure. I'll stay. The work is interesting.'

'Good. Daddy's calling tonight. I'll tell him you got a job and ... and ... how do you feel?'

'All right.'

'I mean——?'

'Am I nervous about it? Is that it?'

'Oh, everybody's nervous on a new job.'

Are they, Mother? Are they all like me and you and Dad? Does everyone live in a shadow of apprehension? Do they all drain the colour out of life, until everything is a melancholy grey?

'Yes, you're right. Everybody's nervous. But when he calls, you tell him I'm O.K.'

When Jay came in and asked about the job I told him I didn't like my boss. He asked a silly question. He said, 'Does it bother you?'

'Of course it does. I have to work with her. She's the Banquet Manager. She's my boss.'

'Well, see how it goes. If you don't like it, you can quit.'

I was angry at him, for his nonchalance about something so important to me. But I followed him into the bathroom. In the small room, the ether smell from the hospital was strong on him.

He turned on the taps to wash. 'Well, how do you like working?'

'Good. I'm not afraid. Oh, tense. Yes. It's a new job. But I know what's expected of me and I can handle it. I like to talk to people, sell myself over the phone. You know, if Mother weren't here I never could——'

'Look, why do you keep repeating that? She *is* here and you *can* work, so——'

'O.K., O.K. I just want you to know.'

'Know what? That I should appreciate her more?'

'No, it's not that.'

'You sure?'

'Yes. I'm sure.'

He dried his hands slowly, methodically. Then he said, 'I called Doctor Borman today.'

'What did he say?'

Tell me he had no time. No room. Tell me so I won't have to go through the strangeness again; the humbling, the pleading, the begging, the laying bare of self.

'He gave you an appointment for next Monday. Is that O.K.?'

'I have to see Downey on Tuesday.'

'Well, that's all right. You can tell him about it if you want to.' He smiled.

'What's so funny? You think it's funny?' I trailed after him through the hall. 'When I look at him, when I have to tell him I saw another doctor, he'll think I'm a fool.'

'No, he won't. Do you think you're being disloyal? Is that it?'

'Yes.'

He put his hands on my shoulders and I felt the pressure of his palms. 'You're not doing a bad thing. You're trying. And I know how hard it is for you. Don't think you're running out on him. You won't be.'

'No?'

'No. Come on. Let's eat.'

'I can't.'

'Please. Tonight eat with me. Sit next to me.' His hand brushed my hair. 'I love you.'

Monday, January 29

All the hours before this one had no meaning. Every crawling moment of the day was merely a prelude. The building lobby was small and hot and very crowded. Three lifts were in constant motion and the moving numbers on the centre panel winked like little red eyes. I scanned the names beginning with B on the directory board and thought, this is not new. I have done this before, and before, and before. Three times in four months. Looking for the name of a doctor. I am a criminal in a crime against myself. My punishment is search. Search for freedom. There it is. *Doctor Martin R. Borman. 1901.* Letters no bigger or smaller than the rest. Nothing to distinguish him from the other ones, the ones who get the patients who can press and point and say, 'It hurts me right here.' And I, sick in every part of me, have no wounds, no scars, nothing that the stethoscope can find, or the finger, or the slide.

'Going up! Up, please.'

'Nineteen, please.'

'Step to the rear of the car, please. That's all. Next car, please.'

The door to 1901 was open. As I stepped over the threshold a musical chime rang twice. I started and moved. It rang again. Then I realized that there was an electrical connection under the mat. I took a big step over it and sat down on the edge of a small leather sofa, waiting for him to throw open the door and glare at me for making the bells ring.

The small room was very hot. I took off my coat and scarf. It was wet with perspiration.

Why the hell do they keep these places so damn hot? What do they want us to do? Sweat it out waiting, and again inside, and then get pneumonia on the way home? Funny. Haven't been sick for a long time. Slight cold in the hospital and that diarrhœa, but nothing else. And I feel so lousy all the time. Maybe I should get sick. Then I'd take my mind off my mind—crazy talk. You're sitting here babbling inanities— remember Staff at the hospital—so you won't think about the next minute or the next when he'll open that door. Then you'll jump up and stammer, so wrapped in fear that his face and body will swim in front of you, formless and formidable. It's only been two and a half weeks. Can you remember Doctor Lowett? Would you know him if you passed him on the street? And Doctor Downey? Can you visualize his face? Clearly? And all the others. Doctor Manning at State? And that little man, also a doctor, who was kneeling beside you last July in the apartment, when you came out of a near-death to a half-life? There's a hell inside of you. A detailed hell. You keep notes on it. You remember every sight and sound and smell of each day. But not the doctors and their faces. You look at them and see yourself. You——

'Mrs. Kruger?'

'Yes. Yes.' I stood up. My scarf dragged. I picked it up. 'Doctor Borman?'

'Yes. Please come in.'

Big brown chair. Sit down. Look down. Open pocketbook. Get out the paper. Dog-eared now. Carried round so much. Now comes the fear that blinds and numbs and wraps round you like a furry cocoon.

A revolving chair squealed and a pair of long legs pivoted towards me.

Look at him. Let it register for once. Stop shaking and concentrate on seeing.

An unshaded ceiling bulb cast a pool of light on his head.

Faded yellow hair. No. Light brown. Not much left. Pale, heavy brows over baggy eyes. Long thin nose. And moustache. Thick, like the eyebrows, and that same straw-brown, drooping, dipping to the mouth. He looks ... he looks ... like what? I don't know ... sort of ... what? Tired. Tired and dull. Reminds me of a ... an animal. Shaggy, baggy dog. English dog. Middle-aged Englishman. House of Lords.

He leaned back in his chair and folded his hands loosely on his lap. His fingers were long, with prominent joints.

Wears a waistcoat. Not many men. . . . My father . . . but suit's not freshly pressed. Sags at the knees. Skinny kegs. Nice socks. Argyles. Back at the feet again. Better look up. He's waiting.

'Doctor Borman, did my husband tell you about me?'

'Briefly, yes. We didn't go into too much detail.'

Flat voice. No highs or lows.

'I have a paper here. This. I typed everything out.' As he tilted forward to take it I thought, merry-go-round. I'm on a medical merry-go-round. I took out my cigarettes and sat hunched and tense, watching his face.

He reads. You stare. Inhale. Exhale. Breathe so loud in this quiet room. That desk behind him. Terribly messy. Doesn't it bother him?

Lowett's desk was empty. He's still on first page. What is he thinking? Hopeless case? Tragic? Classic?

He turned the sheet over. Then suddenly he groped in his back pocket for a handkerchief and sneezed violently. He blew his nose and said, 'Sorry. I've got a nasty cold. I just can't seem to shake it.' He sniffled, cleared his throat, and continued reading. . . . I felt a strange feeling of relief.

The way the sneeze caught him. How he fumbled for the handkerchief. A psychiatrist with a cold. Maybe he's got an ulcer, too. Or rheumatism, like my father. I looked at his bony hands with protruding joints and at his moustache twitching slightly, and at his eyes, blinking and a little watery. He's tired, I thought, and he's got a cold and baggy eyes and not much hair. He doesn't look too healthy or happy. I like that. I'm not happy, either.

When he finished reading he let the paper rest lightly on his lap. Quickly I reached for it.

'Oh', he said. 'Yes. Here you are. Well, how are you feeling now?'

I was disappointed. Why didn't he talk about it? Ask some questions? It's all there, and it's so important. The hospital, the shock treatments, the fear.

'No good. I'm afraid all the time. Not only of the baby. It's everything. Shoes wearing out. Rain and snow. Nappies. My clothes. I'm all mixed up. Recently I thought of a way I could get some peace, some relief——' I swallowed on a dry throat and in the instant of silence I heard clocks ticking behind me. I turned and saw two of them; a small, plain clock and a large one. A bell-shaped glass housed the entire mechanism. Three golden balls suspended from the face moved back and forth in half-circles. I watched it.

'Pretty, isn't it?' he said.

'It's beautiful.'

'Doesn't keep perfect time, though. I still rely on that old one.'

'What is it called?'

'A four-hundred-day clock. You're supposed to wind it only once a year. You were saying?'

'Oh, yes. Well, it's down here on my sheet. I want to leave my baby and my husband and go away. Go home to my mother's place in New York. Or any place. I don't care. I've got to get relief. But I'm afraid to do it.'

'Why?'

'It's not a nice thing to do, is it? My mother tells me how wrong it is, how sorry I'll be. She keeps asking what happened to the love.'

'I don't hear you. Could you speak a little louder?'

I started again, slowly. 'My mother wants to know where is the love Jay and I were supposed to have. How can I want to leave everything? It has nothing to do with love.' I spread my hands. 'I'm sick. She doesn't understand. Do you understand?'

'Yes.'

'You do? Am I right?'

'No. I don't think so. You're in an anxiety state right now. I would postpone this idea of separation. If, after therapy, you find that marriage is not for you, then you can separate.'

'How much therapy?'

'More than you've been getting. It would definitely be worth while.' The moustache twitched, and he sniffled. I thought he was going to sneeze again, but he didn't. He tilted back in the chair and looked at me.

I like this man. This tired, baggy, saggy man who has a cold. I like him for the way he looks and because he is not vague. He is answering my questions. Tears of gratitude sprang to my eyes.

'Doctor Borman, will I get better?'

'Yes. Definitely. In time.'

'How long?'

Press him. Ask and keep asking.

'I don't know. As I said, I strongly advise intensive therapy. Are you going back down South this summer?'

'I don't know. Jay wanted a residency there. It's waiting for him. But now, because of me, I don't think we'll go. I couldn't take the moving, the change. You know I was so well, so busy down there. Before the baby. I wrote. Short stories. Songs. Musical comedies. I was with an acting group.'

Strange, lost little world. Doesn't belong to me any more.

'You can still utilize your drives creatively. When you feel better you can pick up these activities again.'

Now you've spoilt it. Until this minute I believed in you. I don't

*think you really understand, after all. Don't you see I've got a baby?
How can you expect me to be what I was? He's almost eight months
old and I still can't plan and cook a meal. And you think I can do
something creative?*

'Doctor Borman, it's different now with the baby. Everything
is different. I'm not free. I'll never be free.'

'That's true. But as he gets older he'll need less attention.
And you can write again. You can even write of this experience.'

I shuddered. 'I couldn't. Oh, I kept a diary at the hospital.
I still do. But it's too personal. It hurts too much.'

He spread his fingers out. 'They say that sometimes true
accounts are more powerful than fictional ones because the
author writes from his own experience.'

*How the hell did we get on this? Have so many questions for him.
Why didn't he stick to the facts in my paper . . . wonder what time
it is. Afraid to look at my watch . . . can't turn round to see his clocks.
He'll think I'm anxious to leave. I'm not. For the first time I'm not.
I want to stay, to talk to him.*

'Do you know I can't even concentrate on reading or sit
through a film? I'm on pins and needles. These fears. Will I
always be like this? Nervous. So nervous. Compulsive. No
matter how much help I have with the baby and the housework?'

'Yes. It's very difficult to break a basic pattern, but I think in
time you'll learn how to integrate the baby.'

*He uses technical words. Doesn't talk down to me. Knows I'm
intelligent.*

'I try to stop these fears. With my mind. With my will. But
it doesn't help because I don't know the cause.'

'You can get well without knowing the meaning of these
fears. That is, their exact origins.' He reached for a box of
cough drops on his desk, shook it, and one dropped into his
cupped hand. Then he shook the box again.

'Last one.' He popped it into his mouth and smiled. 'Can't
seem to get rid of this cold and sore throat.'

He dropped the box into an overflowing wastepaper basket
under the desk. The desk was an old secretary. The cubbyholes
were choked with papers and pamphlets. Folders were strewn
about with no semblance of order. I looked at him, sitting there

so relaxed, and at that desk behind him, that messy desk. Suddenly I began to shake.

'Now. Right now. I'm scared.'

'About what?' His eyes narrowed slightly.

'I don't know. That's how it is. I see a face on the street or I read a poster on the bus and all of a sudden I have this nameless fear. Doctor Borman, where do they start? Compulsions in general?'

'Well, it's——'

'At six I was that way. I had a box. I kept my toys in it. I wouldn't let anyone touch the box. My mother told me how she and the maid would clean my room and maybe they'd move it a little bit. Then she'd look out of the window and see me coming home from school. And they'd be scared. Of me. Six years old. If I saw my things disturbed I'd yell and run to the box and try to put every little thing back in place. They were really afraid of me. You know, I think I liked——'

'What? I couldn't hear you.'

'Nothing. Anyway, that's just one of the things I did. What was it, what is it with me?'

'Love and hate can co-exist in a person to a very strong degree. If there's no outlet for these feelings, they're placed on to material things. Compulsions are like safety valves. They let out emotional steam.'

Important, important, but do I understand? Love and hate don't go together, but that's what he's saying. And Lowett, didn't he talk about fearing and hating?

'But . . . but it's not just the compulsions. It's other things that made me sick. I'm not feminine. I can't be a mother. My parents gave me dolls. I never liked them. I played house with the kids because they wanted it. I didn't. I'm trapped at home. I don't fit. They told me to get a job. I did. I started last week.'

'How are you doing?'

'Pretty well. I can handle the work. Any work outside. I know what I can do and can't do. . . . You see, I know myself.'

'Yes, I see.' His mouth worked into a shadow of a smile. Then he glanced at the clocks on the table behind me and stood up. He hitched up his trousers. They hung low on his waist.

He tucked his shirt in under the belt and I looked away, thinking, shirt half out, trousers so baggy. If I had a run or a pimple on my nose I couldn't stand so close to him the way he is to me. He's not embarrassed. Why?

'The time is up?'

'Yes.'

Don't want to go. Want to stay and talk to this man.

I gathered my things, stuffed my cigarettes in my purse, and fumbled with the catch. 'I want to thank you, Doctor Borman. Thank you very much.'

Money. Money. Forgot what Jay said about paying him. How could I forget that? Don't want him to think——

He moved to the door and I followed.

'Can you give me any advice? I mean, anything to do?'

Bet he wants to say, yes, what you can do is write me a cheque.'

'Just what we've talked about here. Time. And patience. And hold off on separating until you've had more therapy. You also have to work on your feelings towards Doctor Downey. That's more important than why you're afraid of shoe leather.'

'Yes. I will. Thank you again.' Impulsively I thrust out my hand and he shook it, then walked with me out to the waiting-room. He nodded to a woman in a nurse's uniform.

I walked carefully over the mat so I wouldn't set off the bell again. As I waited for the lift I felt the accumulated tension of sitting huddled and hunched. But my hands were still. They had stopped shaking. Out in the street I looked back at the building, butting tall against the winter sky. Where was his office? His room? His light?

Mother was waiting at the window as I came up the steps.

'Well, hello!'

'Hello, Mom.'

Want to go right to the bedroom and write down everything he said and think and be quiet and lie down.

'We were waiting for you. Both of us. We were watching the buses go by.' She had Gary in her arms. She jiggled and kissed him.

Why does she carry him round so much? Parade him in front of me? His innocence and beauty. She doesn't have to do that. It hurts me.

'What's the good word?'

'No good word. I mean, it was all right. He's very nice.'

'What did he say?'

'I'll tell you later. I want to wash. Did the nappy man come?'

'Yes. And I folded them. Everything's taken care of.'

'And Jay's supper? It's late. I——'

'The chops are defrosted. The potato is baking. I made a fruit salad. There's chicken soup from yesterday and——'

'That's fine.' My eyes scanned the rooms, looking for disorder and things to be set right again. It's always like this, the instant I step inside the house. Caught in the web of compulsion.

'Any cake?' Jay asked.

'Oh, yes. There's cake.' She hurried from the baby's room. He was half-nappied and his plump little buttocks were creased against her arm. 'Cream doughnuts. In the icebox. The second shelf. I put them there to keep them fresh. They looked so good. I knew you liked them.'

He stood at the side of the table, poured himself a glass of milk, and bit into a doughnut. I sat there smoking, watching him drink and eat.

Why doesn't he say something? Ask about Borman. Show some interest. Doesn't he care that I saw a new doctor today? Maybe he forgot. I wouldn't forget. I hate him.

I followed him into the living-room. He sat in the big red chair, one of the pieces he bought at a second-hand furniture store while I was in the hospital. It sat low on the floor, the arms were wide and flat and stained dark with ground-in grime.

How the hell could he buy that chair? It's ugly. And look at his shoes. They're supposed to be white. He doesn't polish them. And he needs a haircut.

'The baby's almost asleep.' Mother came in and sat on the couch.

'Oh, that body. How I love to hold it and put its nappy on.' She folded her hands and looked at us. Neither of us spoke. 'So what did he tell you?' she asked.

I sat down next to her.

'Did you tell him what you want to do?'

'Yes. You'll be pleased to know he advised against it. You happy?'

She was. I saw it in her face. For just an instant. Then she was aware of the sarcasm in my voice and her mouth tightened. 'Yes. Yes, I'm happy. There's a man . . . a doctor . . . who tells you how wrong it is.'

'He didn't say it was wrong. He just said to wait until I have more therapy. That I'm in an anxiety state.'

'See? That's what we're all telling you.'

'Not Jay. Jay doesn't care.'

He turned round and smiled crookedly. 'Are you putting words in my mouth?'

'No, but it's obvious', I said, bitterly. 'Your whole attitude.'

'What attitude?'

'You're so unconcerned. Why didn't you say something when you came home? You knew I saw the doctor, didn't you? What were you waiting for, Christmas?'

'Maybe. (*That set, stubborn smile on his face. I could hit him.*) Did you like him?'

'Yes, I liked him.' I spoke belligerently, still flushed with anger. 'Very much. He seemed to understand. I mean, he gave me definite answers. And he said I'll integrate Gary in time.'

Integrate. Form into a whole. Become united. Be one with my child. Unnatural me. Has to work on love. Everywoman, anywoman, no crushing weight of terror for them. No guilt. No holding back. They touch their babies and feel joy ripple in their fingers. They feel fulfilment. They reach out with willing arms of love. And I turn my back and beat the walls and wish my baby were never born. I have no love to give. Mother does the holding and feeding and clucking and cooing. I stand in the shadows and try to dredge up a feeling that should be welling from me as water from a spring.

'That's what we've all been saying, you know', Jay said. 'You *will* be able to take over in time.'

'See? See?' my mother said. Her eyes glittered. Was it tears or excitement? 'He said it. He's a doctor! He knows! Time. Just time.'

If I hear that word again, I'll scream.

'You don't believe it, do you?' said Jay.

'I want to. But I can't. I——'

'The main thing. Don't forget the main thing', my mother said. 'He said not to go away. Right? Isn't that right?'

'Yes, YES, YES! I haven't packed a bag, have I? I'm still here. You see me, don't you? (*She searched Jay's face for signs of disapproval. Not of me, but of her. She's so afraid of doing or saying things that excite me. I thought of what I had told Borman about the toy box. But I didn't tell him how I liked to see her scared, how it made me——*) It's all right, Mother. Just don't harp on it, huh? I won't leave. I still want to, but I won't. Forget about it, will you? You embarrass me.'

Borman had put out the fire. The idea of running away in a flight of desperation seemed less dramatic and more childish now. I think he knew that I'm in no condition to organize a solitary life, but he didn't tell me that. He considered my plan. He didn't scoff. He gave me decent answers. Supportive answers. And I need them. So badly.

Jay was watching me. I closed my eyes and saw another man sitting there. He was tall and pale and bony and he had a cold. . . .

Wednesday, January 31

Glad I called up Downey and cancelled yesterday's appointment. It gives me time to think. Three blocks from the hotel is the street where Borman has his office. Each time I pass that corner I can see him, sitting like a ghost above the crowds passing by. Why can't I have him? Why? Why not?

Thursday, February 1

The whole thing started off so innocently. I went to see Jay in the doctors' library. It's the only place we can talk together in privacy. It's not really private, because doctors come in to pick up medical journals and some of them stop to chat with him for a few minutes. But it's better than at home.

He was sitting in that deep leather chair. I was in the tall straight wooden one, balancing an ashtray on my lap. He asked me how I was going at my job, and I said, 'I like it. You know, it's good to get out of the house and work at something I can handle.'

And then he said, 'Maybe you should never have married.'
The words, spoken low, almost without expression, cut the
quiet air.

I flushed. 'Why?'

'You don't seem to want the responsibilities of marriage and
everything that goes with it.'

*So blunt. So sudden. He had never said this before. Even when I was
on my want-to-leave-home jag. What's he been doing? Saving up his
hate? Now he tells me.*

I put out my cigarette, grinding the butt with my fingers.
I was cold now, even in the hot room.

'Jay, do . . . do you remember how you kept telling me three
things? Over and over. You said I love you, you're going to get
well, and it will take time. Remember?'

You didn't forget? You couldn't have. You——

'Yes. I remember.' He slumped deeper in the chair. There
were dark circles under his eyes. His white uniform was creased
and there were two brown spots of dried blood on the front of
his tunic. 'I was trying to encourage you in your anxiety. You
were just out of the hospital. Now——'

'Now what?'

*What do you want from me? Guilt? I have more than enough to spare.
Apologies? I can give you those, too. For disturbing your sleep. For
making you drive to the hospital on your free Sundays. For banging my
head on the wall when you wanted to study. For spoiling your plans for
the residency. You haven't mentioned it for months. You barely talk to
me. I always come to you. Even here, in this room. I'm the one who calls
and asks whether I can come over.*

'I'm tired of holding up a one-sided marriage.'

'But I'm trying! I don't want to break up any more. I don't.
When I saw Borman I realized how hasty it was. How wrong. I
don't want to chuck up everything. I want to stay with you and
work it out. But I need your help. It's hard enough alone. When
you don't help me——'

'Judy, I'm just tired.'

'So am I. All the time. I want to sleep. Drown myself in sleep
for a week . . . a year. Look. Maybe it's the same with you.
These long duty nights. The strain. I love you. Please don't be
angry.'

'I'm not angry. I'm disappointed. And other things . . .' He pressed two fingers on his forehead. 'All right, maybe I'm just over-tired. I don't know.'

'Doctor Kruger—Doctor Jay Kruger', the inter-com rasped.

He walked to the wall telephone and flipped the switch. 'Doctor Kruger. Yes. All right. I'll be there.' He buttoned the collar of his tunic. 'I've got to go.'

'Yes. I heard. Jay?'

'It's an emergency. I'll see you tomorrow afternoon.'

As he walked out of the door he nodded to another intern. They walked away together. I imagined them talking.

'*Hi! Quiet on your ward tonight?*'

'*Pretty good. What's new?*'

'*Nothing much. Just told my wife I'm sick of our marriage. She's been ill. A breakdown. Just because she had a baby. Eight months now. I've got it up to here.*'

Friday, February 2

'Doctor Downey, I . . . I have something to tell you.' I was rolling the edge of his appointment card between my fingers. Now it was soft and wet. 'I have a job.'

'That's fine.' He smiled. 'How are you getting on?'

'Pretty well. I'm a telephone solicitor for a hotel.'

He frowned in amusement.

'I mean I handle bookings for weddings, meetings, parties.'

I'm not me. I'm Miss Jones. A simple, fictitious name. Neatly anonymous. I'm Miss Jones on the phone and on the booking sheets. I'm a pleasant, impersonal voice talking to strangers. For four hours a day I can hide in peace.

'Oh, yes. I understand. It sounds like interesting work.'

'Doctor Downey, there's something else. Something I did.'

He's still smiling. Wait until I tell him. Feel so small and guilty . . .

'What is it?'

'I saw another doctor. I couldn't help it. I mean, I'm not making headway.' The card crumbled in my hand and the pieces fell to the floor. 'Since I realized I didn't want a baby nothing is moving or changing. I'm not getting better.'

And Jay. It's worse with Jay. I'm so worried . . .

'Who is the doctor?'

'Doctor Martin Borman. A doctor at Jay's hospital recommended him. Are you angry with me?'

Quick. Bend for the papers. Pick all the pieces from the rug. Don't look at his face.

He spoke calmly. 'What is more important is why you're so restless. I feel I'm competent. Your running round to other doctors shows you don't want to get down to therapy with me and to stop relating symptoms. To face yourself and the situation and try to work your problems out.' He leaned back and rolled a pencil between his fingers.

Now I'm getting it. And I deserve it. Yes, I do.

'I'm concerned that you may go from one doctor to another, clutching at straws. You may get involved with a quack or someone who recommends some unproved chemical technique. It happens that Doctor Borman is an excellent man. I know him. But you seem to be looking for immediate concrete answers and explanations for every one of your symptoms instead of buckling down to therapy.'

Buckle down, Winsocki, buckle down . . . you can win, Winsock——

'I want to try and help you see yourself. You go from week to week with me. You're reluctant to make appointments in advance.'

Maybe he's right. Borman said the doctor-patient relationship is more important than anything else. But the symptoms are so strong. And I want sleep. And peace. And to know what happened to me. Maybe I'm hedging. But it's not deliberate. I'm sure it isn't.

He stood up. 'I can't force you to let go of your complaints and start working on yourself in earnest. It's up to you.'

'Do you want to see me again?'

'It's not what I want, Judith. Do *you* want another appointment?'

'Yes', I said.

He leaned over his appointment book. 'How about next Wednesday at three?' His fingers curled round the pencil.

'All right.' He began to write.

I grabbed the arms of the chair and pulled myself up. 'Doctor Downey, don't be angry . . . but . . . could I call Doctor Borman . . . see if he'll take me on? Oh, God, I'm sorry. I mean, I just want to try him. Not on a lark. I won't go from doctor to doctor. I promise. Everything you said is right. But it's a feeling . . . a . . . are you angry?'

He put down the pencil, closed the book, and stood up. He was so tall beside me. 'No. Why should I be? Do whatever you think you want. He's a very good doctor. Let me know how you make out.'

I followed him to the door, my body sagging and my coat crushed against my chest. I felt small and dirty and evil. 'I'll let you know, Doctor Downey—I will. Thank you for everything. I know how you tried. It's me. It's my fault.'

'Good luck, Judith.'

'Thank you. I'll call you.'

He smiled. Tears choked my throat and eyes. Tears of shame, of gratitude, of relief.

'How did it go today?' Jay asked.

'What?'

Give him a dose of his own medicine. Give him the three C's. Cool, Calm, Collected.

'I said, how did it go?'

'What do you want to know?'

'What's wrong with you?'

'Nothing. Nothing at all.'

'Look, I'm sorry. Those things I said. I've been feeling crummy. Terribly tired. And I'm worried about you and us and the future. (*That's fine. A nice excuse. Why didn't you say something like that before? You think so much more than you say, Jay. You store things in secret places of your mind. You hold yourself in. So different from me.*) Where's your mother?'

'She went out to post some letters.'

He got up and sat down next to me on the sofa. Then he turned my face and kissed me on the mouth, gently.

'Sweetie, I'm sorry. I shouldn't have said what I did. You're having the worst of it. I know you are.'

'Why did you kiss me?'

'Because I felt like it. Don't you want me to kiss you?'

'Yes, but——'

Doesn't follow. First he's cruel, then he—— Not logical. Upsets me.

13

'You think I'm cold, don't you? No heart. No sympathy.'

'No. It's just that . . . well, a few nights ago you said——'

'That was a few nights ago. Can't I change?'

No. Doesn't he know I can't cope with change? In anything. Or anyone.

'Not about something like that. Not when you say you're sick of me and this marriage. You're mean and unfair and you're not helping me. *Now* why are you smiling?'

'I'm glad to hear you talk like that. Telling me how you feel.'

'I've been doing that all the time. I'm a pest.'

'No, you're not. Anyway, right now you're speaking truthfully. I hurt you and you hate me for it and you're right. And I'm sorry. I had a mad on. I got over it. I don't feel that way now.'

I made no reply.

'I won't leave you. I promise. You'll get well. It may take longer than I thought, but everything's going to be O.K. With us and the baby. Do you believe me?'

'All right. I believe you. But I get so scared when you talk like you did that night. Like a hole opening up right in front of me. Another emptiness. Another fear. I need you so much. I don't think you know——'

'I do.' He took my hand and patted it. 'Now tell me what happened with Downey today.'

'I broke with him. Told him about Borman. I was so scared. But he wasn't angry. Then he told me that I harp on symptoms and won't get down to real therapy.'

'Maybe he's right. He's a good man.'

'I can't help it. It's nothing deliberate. When he started to give me another appointment I felt as though a trap were closing. I told him I wanted to ask Borman to take me on. He told me to go ahead.'

'If you want Borman, ask him.'

'I will. I felt so good with him. So right. It's hard to explain. As if I've been running and running and then I came home.'

'When will you call him?'

'On Monday. After work.'

'Want some milk and cake, sweetie?'

'No. No, thanks.'

Wouldn't go down. Lump in the chest.

When Mother came in her cheeks were flushed.

'Cold out, huh?'

'Yes. But I love it.'

'You didn't even have a scarf.'

'I wasn't cold. You know me. I like to walk. I like the air.'

'Mom, don't you get restless here? You never get a chance to go out . . . or . . . go home.'

'What's home? The furniture sticks? The splinter floors? They'll be there when I get back.'

'What about Dad?'

'Will you stop worrying about him? You get well. That's the most important thing.'

'I bet you never dreamed you'd have to stay with me. When you came down South——'

'No, I didn't. But what's the difference? Nobody knows what's going to happen.'

'But it has been long, hasn't it? You admit it?'

'There's nothing to admit.' She wriggled out of her coat. Her eyes were guarded and suspicious. 'What do you want me to say? That I miss Daddy and my home?'

'Yes.'

'I'm not dancing in the streets. I'm not here for the happiest reason. But I told you, how I feel is not important.'

'Why not? You have feelings, too.'

'Sure. I got feelings. I feel I'm here because I'm needed. At least I hope I'm needed.' She flung her short arms out like wings. 'And why the third degree? Did something happen tonight? With you and Jay?'

'No. Nothing.'

'You sure?'

'Yes.' I followed her to the hall closet. She slipped out of her coat and wrapped a housecoat round herself. 'Mom?'

'Yes, dear?'

'I'm sorry. All those questions I asked. I didn't mean to put you on the spot.'

'That's all right. You want some coffee? Milk?'

'No.'

'So go to bed. Get some sleep.'

I bent to kiss her. The hollow of her cheek was soft and dry and smelt musk-sweet. 'G'night, Mom.'

'G'night, darling.'

Why am I and why is she? Why doesn't she complain? Look at her, standing there. So strong. I can't stand her strength, her sacrifice, her giving, giving, giving. She shames me. I hate her. Want to hurt her. With questions. And digging. And when I do I'm sorry. Sorry because she's my mother and I love her. There's no end. Just no end.

Monday, February 5

Dammit, dammit, dammit. Middle of the city. A million stores. A million places. So I had to walk into this restaurant. All day long, I'm dialling his number in my mind. Waiting for him to answer. Waiting, waiting. So the goddam booths in the hotel lobby have to be filled . . . if I go home Mother will hear me . . . and where the hell are the phones in this damn place? So noisy. So many people. Look at those fat pigs pushing their trays along with their bellies. Can't stand this smell of food.

I spoke to an attendant wiping off one of the front tables. 'Any phones at the back, please?'

'No. We got 'em up here. See?' She pointed to the wall. Four open telephones were lined up against the tile wall.

Great. No privacy. People all round. Not even a shelf for my pocketbook. Sweating in this heavy coat. Why the hell did I wear it today? Maybe I should find a—no. Do it now. Here. Or you'll never do it.

I pulled off my earrings and jammed them into my pocket. Then I took out a dime, a pencil, and the slip of paper with his number on it. As soon as I touched it the paper became wet.

Now get over there and call him. Remember. Talk low. They're all round you. They can hear you.

I dropped my pocketbook on the floor and put my foot on it.

They're not going to steal from me. Have to bend the mouthpiece down. Somebody tall used this before me. Tall and dirty. It's full of grease and smells bad . . . dial. Easy. Carefully. No mistakes. Ringing now. Once. Twice . . . answer me, please. . . . Three ti——

'Hello.'

'Doctor Borman?'

'Yes?' His face floated on the white tile wall.

'This is Judith Kruger. I saw you on January 29th. A consultation.'

'Oh, yes.'

'Doctor Borman, I was very impressed. I mean, I got a lot out of it. I liked you. (*This is agony.*) Could you take me on as a patient?'

'I'd have to charge you fifteen dollars a session.'

Right away money. Why didn't he say, sure, if you want me . . .

'That's all right. I'm working part-time. My husband . . . we talked it over. It's all right.'

'Have you discussed this with Doctor Downey?'

'Yes. I told him I wanted to try——'

'When can you make appointments?'

A tray crashed behind me and a spoon hit my ankle. A puddle of soup crept along the floor. I had to drop the receiver and grab up my pocketbook.

'Hello?' I heard his voice at my knees.

'Yes. I'm here. Something spilled. I'm in a restaurant. What did you say?'

'About appointments.'

'Any afternoon.'

'Just a minute. Looks as though I can't see you until Thursday . . . no, Friday. February 9th. At five-fifteen.'

'That's all right. I'll be there.'

'See you then.'

'Thank you, Doctor Borman. Thank you very much. Good-bye.'

I cradled the receiver gently.

Over. All over. Wasn't so bad. He could have been more cordial, though. Downey sounds nicer on the phone. Warmer. Did I make a mistake? Maybe I've built him up too much and too high. Four days to wait. To make sure my feeling was right. Look at this mess on the floor. Why don't they clean it up?

Then I saw two white-coated attendants, carrying mops and pails, weaving through the tables. Their faces were dull and impassive. Suddenly the room blurred and panic, the old panic, pressed in on me. The rumble of voices rose to a roar. I was back in the hospital. In the cafeteria. I had had a seizure.

No, not me. The woman over there. She fell and knocked my tray to the floor. Now they're mad and they're coming after me with sticks in their hands and they'll put me in the room with bars. You, over there. And you. You're my friends, aren't you? Stop them. Hide me. Have to hide. Run and hide. Why can't I run?

I ripped off my glasses and ground my fists in my eyes. When I pulled them away the voices and the faces were gone.

'Excuse me, miss. We got to get in here.'

'Oh, yes. Sure.' I stepped away from the mops and put my glasses on.

Everything was back in focus, clear and undistorted. What happened to me? Am I having a relapse? Or hallucinations? Why now? Why this minute and in this place? What had I been thinking of? The appointment. Waiting for the appointment. Breaking with Downey. The change. Big step. Giant step. Remember that game? . . . you may take two giants . . . Small then. Six or seven. A child. Jumping pavement lines. Getting closer to the leader. Have to touch him to win. And then run away.

'Mother, I called up Doctor Borman today. Do you remember him?'

'Yes. Of course I do. You liked him, didn't you?'

'Yes. I asked him to take me on as a patient.'

'Oh. Well, what about Doctor Downey? Is it all right by him?'

Don't yell at her. Answer her nicely.

'Yes, Mother. I told him what I wanted to do. I wouldn't walk out on someone like that.'

'Is Borman better?'

'It's not a question of better. I just think I can make more progress with him. I have an appointment for this Friday after work.'

'Is everything all right there? I mean, the job.'

'It's O.K. I ought to get about six dollars' commission at the end of the week.'

'So what does she say?'

'Who?'

'Your boss. About bringing in the business.'

I laughed at her. 'Mother, I'm supposed to do that.'

'Well, not everyone could sell over the phone. I couldn't. It's
hard.'

'No. It's not hard. Not for me. I told you I know what I can
handle. And I can't handle a baby.'

'Tell that to the new doctor.'

'I did. Remember?'

'So tell him again.'

'Don't push me. I'll tell him what I want to.'

'I'm not pushing. I just said——'

'I don't care what you said. You always make me nervous.'

'What did I say? I'm asking you, what did I say?'

'Nothing. Never mind. I'm sorry. How's the baby?'

'All right. He's ready for sleep. I wanted to take him out
today. Then the sun went in. I had him dressed. He got cranky.
Then the sun went in.'

'You said that.'

'Yes. Well . . .' She sat with her hands in her lap, twisting
her wedding ring.

*Mom, Momma, Mom. What's wrong with us? Why do we always
clash like this? There's love. There has to be love. And there's shame
and guilt for the words that cut and hurt. I'm always hurting you,
aren't I? But is it all my fault? You goad me, you bait me, you trap me.
You don't know it, but you do. With questions, with the set of your
head and the tone of your voice. If I could talk to you about this . . .
if I could reach you . . .*

'Central Hospital.'

'Doctor Jay Kruger, please.'

'Doctor Kruger speaking.'

'Jay?'

'Hi.'

'That matter we discussed. You know, regarding the change.
I took care of it this afternoon.'

'Good. Good. Glad to hear it. When will it happen?'

'This Friday. But I have to notify the other one. I haven't
done that yet. I'm a little . . . well, it's awkward.'

'I don't think so. This happens plenty of times. I think you're
building it up. No, I didn't mean that. Just take care of it.'

'O.K. When will I see you?'

'Tomorrow night. How's Gary?'

'Fine.'

'O.K., then. I'll see you. G'bye.'

'Doctor Downey?'

'Yes.'

'This is Judith Kruger.'

'How are you?'

'Pretty good. I just wanted to tell you I saw . . . I mean, I spoke to Doctor Borman today. He's willing to take me as a patient.'

'I see.'

'I know we talked about whether it was wise (*my chest is bursting*), but I really felt I want to make a change. You're sure it's all right?'

'Of course. You're free to do whatever you think best.'

Free. Did I free myself from you to blunder again? Was it the right thing? Sound like Mother now. Right thing, wrong thing . . .

'Thank you. I called as soon as possible. In case you wanted to schedule another patient. I think you kept this Wednesday for me?'

'Oh, that's all right. Don't worry about it. Well, lots of luck to you, Judith.'

'Thank you. Good-bye.'

Warm, he was. Not curt or short. And wished me luck. All mixed up again. Why did I leave him? Resistance to therapy, he said. Maybe, maybe, call him back and then call Borman and then . . . Mother again . . . this is what she'd tell me if she were inside me . . . if she knew my fears. No, this is final. Must go to Borman. Must work with him. Can't try or test him or fight him.

Friday, February 9

Those nightgowns in that window. Pretty. Do I need any? Brassières, maybe? Only have four. There's a sweater. Mine are old. Everything's old . . . those belts. What size am I? Can't remember. And hats. Don't have a hat. Should I have a hat . . . don't know what I want . . . want . . . want . . . afraid of these stores. Can't buy things any more. Can't concentrate or decide. It hurts. Really hurts. Feel flat and squashed. I walk like a pygmy among giants, afraid the world will fall on me.

I turned off Walnut Street and entered Rittenhouse Square. Children, bundled against the cold, waddled like little space men along the cement walks, or scratched with sticks in the hard brown earth. An old man on a bench was throwing chunks of bread to the pigeons. They milled round him, swooping and pecking. Nurses in grey capes wheeled expensive baby carriages, manœuvring them past the clusters of children and mothers in slacks. One nurse ducked her head under a cloud of cigarette smoke hanging motionless in the still winter air.

I thought, I'm walking among them. If I told them I was afraid of their children and the pigeons and the smell of winter and the clothes on their backs and the light of living in their eyes. . . . If I told them. . . . You women there, chattering, smoking, wiping runny noses, pushing mittens on tight-fisted hands. You have integrated. Do you know that word? Do you know what it means? You don't have to. You went home from the maternity ward. I went to a mental hospital.

I walked down the wide stone steps to the street. A child's skate lay upturned on the bottom steps, its wheels still spinning. I wanted to kick it until it flew apart. . . .

I was twenty minutes early. I smoked in the ladies' room and thought of my first week's salary. I had made seven dollars in commission, more than I had expected. But that bitch didn't say a word when she handed me the pay envelope. Nothing except 'that McCullough engagement shower cancelled. I knew they would'. As if it were my fault. And no praise for the other jobs I booked. Why is she so mean to me? I hate her.

When I walked into his office I was still five minutes early. That was just right. I didn't want him to think I was too anxious. Oh, no. Not anxious. Merely desperate.

He opened the inner door and the instant I saw him I knew nothing had changed. Not in him. The same stretchy leanness, the faded brown hair, the tired face lines disappearing in the drooping moustache.

He nodded. 'Come in.'

The office was dark. Heavy curtains were drawn across the only window. The standing ashtray by the couch was crammed with cigarette butts. The golden balls in the bell clock turned silently inside their cage.

He sat in the swivel chair next to his desk and steepled his
fingers.

'Well, how are you feeling?'

'Guilty.' I managed a smile. 'About leaving Doctor Downey.
I still feel maybe he was right. About always complaining of
symptoms and not getting down to therapy. I . . . wait a
minute. I want to get a cigarette. (*Stall. No. Don't. You wanted to
come and now you're here and this is costing fifteen dollars a session.
Talk to him. For God's sake, tell him . . .*) Doctor Borman, I have
empathy with you. Is that the word? I think it is . . . a feeling.
It's hard to explain. This may sound crazy. You're not good-
looking (*omigod, he'll hate me for sure, now*) . . . you look human.
Tired. Not so happy. I can't stand people who are happy. I
I feel I can talk to you. A rapport. A sympathy, maybe, I don't
know. It's so hard to explain. You look "Haimische". That's
Jewish. Are you Jewish?'

He nodded and his eyelids flickered briefly.

*I forced him and they don't like to be forced. Patients should know
as little as possible about the personal aspects of their doctors.*

'It doesn't make any difference, really. No. That's not true.
It does make a difference that you're Jewish. I feel better with
you. I shouldn't, but I do. And the first time I saw you. You
gave me concrete advice on separating. Let me ask you something. Why are doctors afraid to give definite answers to their
patients? Sometimes they need it. I do. You told me I'll get
well. I believed you. You told me I'd learn to integrate. I hope
so. You know, I feel funny sitting here. It's hard to believe I'm
a psychiatric patient. It's always been other people. In books
and films. Someone else. Now me.'

'Are you sleeping any better?'

'No. I've tried everything. Nothing works on me any more.
When I took those sleeping pills before I went to the hospital
I think I swallowed eight or ten. Maybe more. And I only
slept for two hours. It shows you how nervous I was. Oh, I'm
better now. But always tense and afraid. And the nights are so
bad. Things go round and round in my mind. If I could only
shut off my brain and get some sleep.'

He reached over to the back of his desk and picked up some
small bottles. 'Here. Try these. Take three for three or four

nights. Then switch to these—the large ones. Your husband has them?'

'He can get them. (*If Jay wasn't a doctor . . . oh, God, the drugstore bill!*) What was that again? Three of these?'

'I'll write it down for you.' He tore off a sheet from a scratch pad.

I must do that too. Write it down. Everything he tells me. Can't do it here. Patients can't take notes in a psychiatrist's office. That's crazy. I'll do it down in the lobby. As soon as I leave him.

'Doctor Borman, you said I could get well even if I don't know the origins of my fears and phobias?'

'Yes.' He nodded and sniffed and his moustache twitched.

Definitely like a dog. Big, shaggy. Relaxed. Yet awake and listening.

'But they must have meaning. Shoe leather. Things out of place. Holes in clothes.'

'They do have meaning. But they're only a small part of a larger picture. If you should gain insight into a particular set of obsessions, that still won't prevent another type cropping up in the future. (*So what's the good? If he helps me find out why I'm scared of holes, maybe I'll start in with something else. Like washing my hands twenty times a day.*) . . . patient relationship.'

'What? I'm sorry. I was thinking of something.'

'What was it?'

'Nothing.'

If I told him every little thing that crosses my mind we'd never get anywhere.

'I said it's more important to work on our relationship.'

Our relationship. Sounds dirty. Or loving.

'You mean how I react to you? Why?'

'Because the way you act and talk to me shows your attitudes to other people and situations.'

'And that's important?'

'Very.' He smiled and the lines in his face relaxed.

'All right, but . . . but what can I do about my compulsions? It's not fear that I don't believe you, but they're so pressing. And the fear. Why am I so tense? It's not only the baby. It started with him, but it's spread.'

'I think the emotional shock of childbirth triggered these fears. They were probably always there.'

I thought of Dr. Lowett when he said the birth trauma had broken down my defences. 'Can you help me? Give me some advice? On these compulsions?'

'Right now I'd suggest you force yourself not to give in. Do something more constructive to release energy and tension.'

'Sometimes, on the way to the kitchen to make supper I— my mother makes it, really. I just stand round and wring my hands. Anyway, I see dust on the windowsills in the living-room. And I want to get water and a sponge and wipe the dirt away. That's wrong?'

'At that particular time, yes. Try to force your eyes away from the dust and go on to the kitchen.'

'I can tell you right now that's hard. Very hard. I feel better when I do what I have to do, and right away. I feel safe, sort of.'

He nodded. 'I understand. But you try it. Try to tolerate the anxiety and go on to a more realistic task.'

This is important. Have to write all this down.

'Doctor Borman, I still feel it's a mistake. A terrible mistake. Me having a baby. And I thought I wanted it so much. It was a compulsion. Like everything else. And now it's over and I'm sick and I'm trapped.' I thumped the chair with my fist.

'Yes. I understand that.'

'Do you? Really?'

Do you know what it's like to have steel bands in your chest, crushing and squeezing you with guilt?

'Even though you recognize the mistake, so-called, and you say you're not maternal, you should try to change your attitude. Try to accept him.'

'I can't believe I had him. No. That's not true. I don't want him. And that's why I hate myself so much.'

'There are many women who feel very little attachment for their child in the early months. As the baby grows and you establish a more intellectual relation with him, you feel closer.'

Great! Do I have to wait until my son and I can talk politics together? I'll be dead by then.

He shifted himself in the chair. 'Of course, there is a possibility that when you start to care for him on your own, you may have a recurrence of the anxiety. But you'll know how to control the symptoms better. You'll be all right.' He smiled.

'I will? Are you sure?'

'You will be able to handle him on your own without a relapse.'

'I feel better when you say that. I feel——'

He's holding me up. I'm leaning on him. Believing him. Anything he says . . .

'What are you doing with yourself?'

'Nothing. Just working. And worrying. That takes a lot of time.' He laughed. It was more like a chuckle, low and rumbly.

Glad I made him laugh. At me. With me. Makes no difference. As long as he likes me.

'Well, something besides that. Have you picked up your writing or dramatics?'

He harps on that. Why? I'm just a few months out of the hospital. Can't cook a meal or buy hair grips in the five and dime without getting the shakes. Wonder if he really understands my case after all?

'I can't. I'm too nervous.'

'Well, it's something to consider for the future.'

'Yes. (*Get him off that subject. Hurts to think about it.*) Doctor Borman, you said that all my compulsions . . . all the things that bother me . . . they're parts of a whole. What do you mean?'

'I don't know. Yet. There seems to be an emphasis on things. Possessions.'

'It's not only things. I'm afraid to travel. Big trips. Moving. And rain and snow and winter. Cold and wetness scare me. I never was like this. What are you smiling about?'

'Do you think I'm smiling?'

Oh, brother—here we go! Typical psychiatric approach. Answer a question with another question. Patient says, 'Hello, how are you?' Doctor counters with a 'Why?' Patient says, 'I just said hello.' 'You just said hello?' 'Yes. Is something wrong?' 'Do you feel it's wrong?' Exit patient, cutting paper dolls.

'It looked as though you were smiling.'

'Perhaps these fears . . . even about the weather . . . aren't new ones. Merely extensions of your obsession with things. Now they've cropped up because you have less control over the anxiety.'

'You mean my nervousness.'

'No. General anxiety, which you've been siphoning off into compulsive acts.'

'I forgot something else. Song rhythms in my head. Senseless repetition of words and phrases. Sometimes I feel like a needle stuck in a record groove. It started in the hospital after I came out of the depression. When I'm busy working it subsides a little. But when I walk through the streets alone, or when my mother goes shopping and leaves me, or late at night when it's so quiet and I can't sleep. . . .'

'What are they like?'

'A repeating and repeating. Like a drum beat. If I hear a commercial on the radio or my mother sings a little song to Gary . . . the rhythm goes on for hours. Sometimes I want to bang my head open.'

'They're all significant.'

'Freud said that about slips of the tongue, didn't he? Is this the same?'

'Essentially, yes.'

'I can't believe it. They're not songs from my childhood. Or things that people said to me. They're senseless. No words. Just rhythms. And that's supposed to have meaning?'

'Sometimes.'

Got him. Stumped him, and he knows it, and he's trying to wriggle out. I'll let him go this time.

'There are other feelings, too. Strange ones. Almost eerie. I look at a radio or a dish or a table and they start to grow.'

'Grow?' His heavy brows puckered.

'Not in size. In impact. (*Said that wrong. He must think I'm really psychotic. Having hallucinations.*) Before I was sick, objects were, well, just there. They occupied space. They didn't intrude on it. Now they seem to push out at me with the very state of their being. Then I'm afraid of them and want to withdraw. What is it? Do you know?'

'Yes. It's fairly common with compulsives. A phenomenon of perception. An intense preoccupation with inanimate things.'

I hunched over. 'But . . . but if I'm so concerned with things, why do I get panicky when I have to shop? Wouldn't you think I'd like to buy and——?'

He touched a finger to his moustache and smiled. 'I think the Greeks had a word for it. "Possess not lest ye be possessed." Compulsive individuals are really afraid to acquire things because the act of possession will consume them. They'll have to worry about everything they own. And no one likes to involve himself in an anxiety situation.'

'Oh, yes. I see what you mean. (*Hated to lend my toys . . . and books . . . and clothes . . . couldn't trust them to take care of my things the way I would . . . they didn't . . . couldn't care as much as I . . . remember . . . 'Judy, could I wear that green sweater of yours tonight, huh? it's so pretty . . . goes with my slacks . . . you know that new counsellor . . . it's my night off tonight . . . he's taking me to the cinema in town . . . could I have it, just for tonight? . . . What? Do I have shields? No. I . . . Well, O.K., I'll pin them in if you got a pair to lend me . . . yes, sure I promise . . . I won't lose it. I'll bring it to the mess hall first thing in the morning . . .'*) Doctor Borman, in the hospital—when I first came—I wanted to be naked. I couldn't look at—I didn't even wear my own clothes. I didn't know why. Now . . . with what you've told me . . . I . . . think I understand . . . a little . . .'

It was hard for me to talk. I was flushed and quivering. As I talked to him I was talking to myself: *I see, I can see . . . He's right. He's smart. He knows. Ties it in. Makes it fit. Feel crazy-light. Such a little thing. Yet . . .*

'It's a vicious cycle, isn't it? I mean, a person like me. I really don't want to possess, but when I have possessions I get so wrapped—or trapped—in them.'

'Yes. Well, that's typical of compulsives. The emotional involvement with things rather than personal relationships. (*He's got me labelled, tagged, and ticketed. Manic? No. Schizoid? Sorry. Nobody here but us compulsive-obsessives.*) That's why having a baby can be such an upsetting experience.'

'What should I do?'

'Do what I told you. Try to accept your baby. Tolerate the anxiety of your compulsive drives and——'

'You make it sound so easy. It's——'

'I know.' He smiled again and nodded his head. 'For the rest of your life you're going to have to fight unhealthy concerns and develop new responses to daily living.'

He tilted forward in his chair and stood up.

'Is it time?' I asked.

'Just about.'

Nuts! I watch his eyes and he watches the clock. Does it so smooth and neat, too. They're all alike. You plunge deep. You think they're with you. All the way. But they're not. Suppose I said, 'Oh, by the way Doctor, I killed my mother last night.' He'd come back with a 'I'm sorry, the hour is up.'

He rustled the pages of his appointment book.

'I seem to be pretty well filled this coming week. I can see you next Wednesday. And we'll work out a twice-weekly schedule. All right?'

'All right. The same time?'

'Yes.'

When I collected my clothing I said, 'Doctor Borman, about the fee. I still owe you for that first consultation.'

'We can forget about that. You're on regular therapy now.'

'Do you want a cheque for this session?'

He ran his fingers through his thin, light brown hair. 'Why don't you pay me monthly? It makes my book-keeping easier.'

'O.K. (*Look at the desk. He keeps records there?*) I'll keep a record.'

'You don't have to. I'll have it marked.'

'But then I'll know exactly.'

'If you want to.'

He held open the door for me. My coat brushed his arm.

'Oh! I'm sorry.' I crushed the coat against my chest.

Mustn't touch him.

'That's all right. See you next week.'

Walking to the bus, a new rhythm pattern developed. 'Not easy . . . not easy . . . the rest of your life . . . rest of your life . . .' Soon my steps matched the inner beat . . . 'sentence from the judge . . . rest of my life . . .' Oh, hell . . . it's not hard, really. Just give yourself a shake, shake, shake and turn yourself about. What? Don't know where to begin? At the beginning, of course. First you break down and then you build up, see? How long? You heard the man. For the rest of your life . . . rest of your li—

Saturday, February 10

We didn't hear him come in. When the inner door clicked shut we both started and crashed into each other.

'It's Daddy!' Mother pressed forward, and then, when she was close to him, a mask of control spread over her face. I hung back. 'Hello, Daddy.' She turned her face so that he could kiss her on the cheek.

'Darling dear', he said. 'You all right?'

'Fine. Fine.'

Then he came over to me. His coat and face were cold from the night air. His eyes were bright and anxious, searching my face for a sign. Without knowing why, I turned my face the way she did. His lips brushed my cheek.

'Hello, Dad.' I avoided his eyes.

'Hello, darling. How are you?'

'Fair. Pretty good.'

'She started with a new doctor', Mother said. 'She likes him.'

'Mother, can I talk, please? I'm not dumb, you know. And let him get his coat off, for God's sake. He just came in.'

They gave each other sharp glances.

'Daddy, come', she said. 'I got kasha. He loves kasha.'

'Did you eat, Mommy?' he said.

'Before. So how are you?' Her eyes narrowed in scrutiny.

Before, before, she always eats before and after and never with him and never with us. And he always asks the same questions. And plays the game of Alphonse and Gaston. 'Taste it . . . no, you taste it . . . it's good . . . eat more . . . I got plenty . . . you sure? . . . I'm sure . . . so sit down and have some . . . I tasted it before . . . no, no more, Mommy . . . all right, just one . . . you sure you ate? . . . yes, I ate . . . so sit with me' . . . Remember the chair? The empty chair. He always made us drag in another chair for her. And she'd stay by the stove and mix and stir and serve and never sit down in that chair. And still he'd make us bring in that damn chair. It gave me the creeps. Like a memorial for the dead.

'I'm fine, Mom. Know what I did?' His shoulders shook in childish excitement. 'I made my bed this morning!'

'No!' Mother laughed.

'Shah, shah!' He shushed us with a wagging finger. Then he

14

took off his coat and moved with little mincing steps towards Gary's room. 'Aren't you forgetting someone? The most important one in this place here? How's my boobala?' He clapped his hands to his head. 'Oy, oy, oy! Is that sweet? I dream about him. I talk to his picture. You know, the one before the bath. With his business sticking out.'

'Don't ask', Mother said. 'Don't ask. Guttenu, how I love him. A thousand times a day I eat him up. Tonight he fell asleep like a doll. Yesterday he——'

'Mommy, tell me, how can I wait until the morning?' He peeked round the side of the cot and sighed.

'Come eat now. I got everything ready.'

'O.K., Mommy. Let me wash a little.'

The bathroom door was open. I walked in as he was washing his hands, his body hunched over the sink, and his palms cupped to catch the water.

'Hi', I said.

'Oh, darling. I didn't hear you.'

'You O.K., Dad?'

'Fine. Little tired, that's all.'

'How's everything at home?'

'Fine.'

'You eating O.K.?'

'Sure. What are you, worried about me or something?'

'No, no.' I waved my hand. 'I just . . .'

Sure, I'm worried. Pity-worry. Guilt-worry. I'm leaning on every-body. Pulling and sucking from them. Upsetting their lives.

He was rubbing his hands briskly. 'Darling? Something wrong?'

'No. You'd better go in. Mother has supper for you.'

'So how about you?'

'I'll have something later. Anyway, you want to talk.'

'What talk? We have secrets or something?'

'I didn't mean that.'

'Say, what's this about a new doctor?'

'Yes. I'm seeing someone else now.'

'Why? The other guy was no good?'

'No. I just wanted to make a change.'

'Is this one a good doctor?'

'Yes. Very. But the important thing is how the patient feels towards the doctor. I feel——'

In a sudden movement he grabbed my hands in his. 'And that pussy-doll inside there isn't important? Honey . . . darling . . . how can you be afraid of him? He's so good . . . he's so innocent . . . he——'

'Dad! Please!' I pulled my hands away. 'Leave me alone. You don't understand. It's not the baby. It's me. Me!' I punched my chest with my fist. 'I'm sick and I'm abnormal and I know it, so leave me alone!'

Mother ran to the doorway. 'What happened? What happened?'

He whirled, fear in his eyes. 'Nothing. I was just . . .' Then his face set in a pout. 'Now don't yell, Mommy. Don't yell.'

'It's not his fault', I said.

'Come on in the kitchen', she said.

'O.K., Mom. Sure. Sure.'

When I went to the bathroom at one in the morning I heard them talking. Her voice hissed and his voice whined. He sounded like a child.

Wednesday, February 21

Why the hell does it rain every time I have an appointment? Hate to drag all these wet clothes into his office. But I can't leave them here, in the waiting-room. Somebody could walk in and steal them. Clothes, clothes, clothes, always worrying about my clothes . . . possess not lest ye be possessed . . . wonder what kind of people live in nudist camps . . . do they shed their clothes to get close to nature or because they don't want to be bothered . . .

A thread of water from my boots snaked across the wine-coloured rug.

Looks like I'm bleeding. Or urinating. Now, why do I think like that? Morbid and dirty.

'Hi.'

'Hello, Doctor Borman.'

Cheeks burn. Throat goes dry. The first moment is always the worst. With him, and Jay, and my father . . . and so many others. The sudden fear . . . a turning in . . . a feeling that I want to hide . . .

'Come in', he said.

'Yes. But . . .' I pointed to my boots. 'Your rug . . . I got it wet. I couldn't help it. It's——'

'Oh, that's all right. Don't worry about it.'

I watched him settle himself. He swivelled his chair down low, stretched his legs and crossed them at the ankles, and hooked his thumbs under his belt.

I thought, Doctor Downey put his feet up on the desk. Doctor Manning at the hospital flung one leg over the chair arm. What's with them? Why must they spread and sprawl like that? Exhibit their maleness. A woman can't do that. She must keep her feet together and her skirt down. If she crosses her legs it must be discreetly. They have so much freedom . . .

'Well, how are you?'

'Existing.' I puckered my mouth.

'Is that all?' He smiled.

'Going from day to day.'

'Well, that's something. How's the job?'

'The same. The commission isn't bad. I never worked for commission before.'

'Do you like it?'

'Yes. It makes you work a little harder. (*This small talk is costing me money. Fifteen dollars divided by fifty. How much is that a minute?*) Doctor Borman, I really appreciate the information you gave me about my compulsions. You know, when I left here last time I summarized all the things we talked about and wrote them down so I'll remember.'

'You don't have to remember everything I tell you.'

'I feel safer.'

'I imagine you do.'

'It's like you're the teacher and I'm the student.'

'You liked the teachers who were explicit? Who outlined the lesson?'

'Yes. Very much.' I smiled. 'I hated the ones who rambled with no form or order. They didn't give me anything concrete.'

'Concrete. The substance . . . it's strong, isn't it? But it's rigid. Unyielding.'

'I know. And I know I have to pigeon-hole facts. But it's the only way I can learn.'

'Well, as time goes on, I think you'll be able to develop new patterns that have more spontaneity. And you, yourself, will become less rigid.'

'I hope so. God, I hope so. But this rigidity, and the compulsions, and the . . . what was it you said, the involvement with things instead of people . . . it's nothing new . . . it came from way back, didn't it . . . I mean, my parents, the way they raised me? Particularly my mother. I don't want to put the blame on her.

Ho, ho! you don't? Like hell you don't! You want to get off the hook and hook her. And she's the most logical . . . the most vulnerable . . .

He tipped back in the chair and rolled his tongue under his lip. The thick moustache did a little dance. 'I think it's a combination of environment and the person's constitutional make-up. The individual is like a seed. The environment is the soil. Environment is only half the story. You have to face yourself as you are and——'

'——change', I broke in. 'First accept. Then adjust. Is that it?'

'Precisely.' His head bobbed.

Now he really sounds British. Wonder if he's got a snuff-box? Maybe pushes a pinch up his nose and sneezes between patients . . . now I'm making fun of him. Said hello a few minutes ago with such humble eyes. These mood changes of mine . . . can't understand them . . .

'Look, since I mentioned my mother . . . I want to tell you something. She hovers over the baby so much it makes me nervous. We're all sitting in the living-room, see . . . she gets up . . . she goes to his room. She puts her hand in the crib to feel for a draught. And outside in the street. She's always turning the pram to get out of the wind. And when she feeds him, she'll stand on her head, almost, to get the food into him. When I say, "Mother, that's enough. He doesn't want any more', she says 'All right, but maybe one spoon more." And then I get so tight and angry inside I could almost hit her.'

'Why?'

'Just what I told you. Because she hovers and worries about him so much. More than I worry.' My hands tightened on the arms of the chair.

Think. Think. There's more. Reason behind the reason. Feel it. Drag it out.

'More than I *want* to worry . . .' I leaned back and thought,
this is like labour—a bearing down and squeezing out. 'I
don't want my baby and I don't want to get involved with it the
way a real mother should . . . the way my mother does . . . I
hate her because she cares more than I care . . .'

'Do you remember what you told me about the interview
with Doctor Lowett?'

'Y-yes. I think so. He said a new mother tries to outdo her
own mother in caring for her baby. And a rivalry develops.'

'Exactly!' He sat up now, his hands on his knees. 'An undeclared war to determine who is doing more for the child's
welfare. Basically, I think *that* is the root of your feelings, and
not so much the fact that you don't want the baby.' He leaned
back.

I studied the floor and remembered Lowett's pomposity, his
brusqueness, and my confusion and anger.

I spoke low. 'So he was right?'

'Yes. I think so.'

We sat there in silence. The room was wrapped in twilight.
He reached up, switched on the overhead light, and sat back
again.

'Would you mind? I mean, the light is glary. My eyes are
sort of tired.'

He snapped it off again.

*Not the eyes. The inside. Want to stay dark inside and think . . .
and think . . . is it possible . . . this rivalry thing . . . sounds silly
. . . and yet . . . what did he call it? . . . undeclared war . . . fight
for right . . . who is right . . .*

'You know . . . my mother . . . she's a stickler for the right
thing . . . she's so afraid she won't make a right decision . . .
buying clothes or furniture. Or presents for people. She has
to be right and proper. . . . If she made a wrong decision we'd
never hear the end of it.'

'How did you feel about that?'

'Annoyed. *First* I'd try to calm her. Then I'd get angry and
yell. I couldn't stand her indecision . . . the way she had to see
sixteen sides to every situation. She took the joy out of everything. She——'

I put my hand to my mouth. 'I shouldn't be talking like this.

She's living with me. She takes care of my baby. She cooks for Jay. If it weren't for her. . . . Sitting here, talking like this about her, I feel as though I'm stabbing her in the back. And don't ask me if I *want* to stab her in the back! I know your loaded questions!'

He laughed. 'I won't.'

'You know something? I'm telling you all the things she did that annoyed me and I'm just like her. No kidding. I am. Before I was married she was the boss of the house. I didn't have any decisions to make. The home was her responsibility. Then, when I married, on my own . . . I did everything that she did. I made meat patties just the way she did. I cooked chicken just as she did. I used the same kind of rags and polish to clean house as she did at home. There's nothing wrong in that—I mean, lots of girls do things the way their mothers did. You have to learn from someone. It's just that . . . I felt guilty.'

'About what?'

'If I did anything different from what she did . . . or bought something she'd never buy . . . I felt as though she were watching me and didn't like it. She was hundreds of miles away, but I still had that feeling. Crazy, huh? I'd be buying a birthday present for someone and I'd stand at the counter and finger the things and I'd wonder if Mother would think it was too cheap. I'd try new recipes. If they turned out well I'd send them to her. But I'd write to her "you cream the butter" even though I used margarine. She never used margarine. She always said butter gives a better flavour.'

Tired again. Every time I dig inside I get so tired. This is work. Hard work. I could climb a mountain with greater ease.

I leaned back in the chair. 'You see. It's little things like that . . . I wasn't free. If she could hear me now she'd say, "No, no, no. You're wrong, Judy. Remember how independent you were . . . no one could tell you anything . . . you were such a definite person . . . I always admired you for that." Oh, yeah. That's what I thought, too. I didn't know . . . lots of things I didn't know . . .'

My eyes closed for an instant. I blinked and said, lazily, 'Right now I could fall asleep on your couch.' I pointed to it and then looked at it and suddenly the brown leather looked dirty and the words were dirty. Your couch, your couch, your couch. I shivered and sat up, grabbing for my purse that slipped off my lap.

'I . . . er . . . I raked my mother over the coals, didn't I? I.might as well tell you something about my father. When he came to Philly last Saturday night he——'

His eyes flicked to the clock and he came forward in the chair. 'Suppose we hold that for next session.'

'Is it time?'

'Yes.' He switched on the light and studied his appointment book. 'I can't see you until next Friday. I'm sorry. This month has been very tight. And it'll have to be late. Is that all right?'

'Yes. (*Hate him when he watches that clock. But want to see him more and more. Week and a half until the next time. What'll happen to me?*) It must be a long day for you, Doctor Borman.'

'Some days. Yes.'

I turned away from him to pull on my boots. If my skirt hiked up I didn't want him to see.

'Are you through for the day?'

'No. I have one more appointment.'

I buttoned my raincoat and picked up my umbrella. 'Well, I'm ready to schlep home.'

He laughed.

Good. I can even get a laugh out of a psychiatrist.

'I'll see you next Friday. Good night, Doctor Borman.'

'Good night, Judith.'

As I closed the door I looked at the couch again. It stretched the full length of the small room. It was long and low and ugly brown. I wondered what had possessed me to think I wanted to lie on it.

Friday, March 2

'How have you been getting on?'

The same. Everything's the same. Even the mess on the desk. Getting used to this room now. And him. And the idea of seeing a psychiatrist. Don't feel so creepy now. Or so strange and awkward.

'I'm doing pretty good. Well, I mean. My English. I'm always correcting my mother and smirking at other people's

mistakes. And then I use bad grammar myself. You know something . . . I just remembered. Grammar was the only subject
I ever failed. Not a full fail. Just an exam. In junior high. I got
a sixty-three. Two points below passing. I had to take a make-up
exam.'

'Were you upset about it?'

'Terribly. I kept staring at that test paper and the number
sixty-three and I couldn't believe it. I was so ashamed. I had
terrific marks in everything else. And there was that girl. Her
name was Phyllis Kaplan. I hated her . . .'

'What happened with the grammar test?'

'Oh, I'm sorry. I'm racing today. I feel a little excited. A little
happy. Oh, not really happy. I can't be happy. But I went for
nine days without seeing you and nothing awful happened.'

'Did you feel something would happen?'

'Yes. Last time. I was scared when you said you couldn't see
me until today.'

'Why didn't you say something? I could have called you in
case I had a cancellation.'

'I was ashamed. You'd think I was a baby.'

'You should have told me.'

'A little thing like that?'

'Yes.'

'But I think of so many things as we talk. Mostly about you.
You have no idea how my mind flits . . . I couldn't bring myself
to tell you——'

'Try it. Little by little. The feelings you have for me minute
to minute are more important than a story you bring me
about something that happened last night or even ten years
ago.'

'That's funny. I mean, strange. I thought childhood
memories were the core of therapy.'

'They're important, yes. But the core, as you call it, is right
here in this room. Our relationship——'

'There!' I interrupted. 'I'll tell you something. You asked me
to. Right?'

'Right.' His moustache twitched. I thought he was trying to
suppress a smile.

'Every time you say "our relationship" I think of . . . of

intercourse.' I rubbed my hands together. The palms were sweating.

'Why?'

'That word relationship. It means closeness. Give and take. Up and back. You're a man. I'm a woman. And so I think of intercourse. That's abnormal, isn't it? To see sex in such a general word?'

'Not necessarily. It's a plausible association.'

'Suppose I heard the word and thought of death—something like that—then it *would* be abnormal?'

'Perhaps, but not—'

'—necessarily', I mimicked him. 'It's like pulling teeth to get an answer from you. No. I take that back. I'm sorry. You *have* answered my questions. That's why I like you.'

'You try to pin me down, don't you?'

'I guess I do. My mother used to say the same thing when I'd press her for an answer. And then she'd start with her million questions and I'd feel squeezed.'

'I think the way you needle me shows hostility.'

'Oh, no, Doctor Borman! I need you. I'm not hostile to you.'

'You can need someone, be dependent on them, and still have hostility. We touched on that last week. Your guilt feelings about your mother. And your resentment over the way she cares for the baby.'

I lowered my head and talked to my hands. 'You're angry at me because I'm a pest.'

'No. Nagging is very common in compulsive people. Is it important to you whether I'm angry or not?'

'Yes. Very. I'm afraid when people get annoyed with me. I get very hurt. And I never forget what they said and how they said it. The impact stays and stays. Just as though they'd slapped me and I could still feel the sting. Mrs. Meredith, my boss . . . I can't handle her. When I'm talking to nice people I have a fine command of language. But she's so cold to me. When she makes a nasty crack I shrivel. I can't think of any words to use against her. And I hate her for being so mean.'

'No one should be mean to you?'

'I wish they wouldn't, but I know it's impossible. It's just that I'm so damn sensitive. Let me tell you this. I think it was a day or so after I saw you on consultation. Jay and I had a fight. Not a big one. A tiff. We were talking in the doctors' library in the hospital. I told him I didn't want to run away any more, or separate, that I wanted to work things out. Then, out of the blue sky he says, "Judy, maybe we shouldn't have married." Just like that. He was always supporting me. Telling me everything would be O.K. . . . I love you, darling, and don't worry and you'll get well. Things like that. I was so hurt. And shocked. As though he'd thrown a wet rag in my face.'

'What happened?'

'Two days later I got up the guts to tell him how nasty he was and he says, "I had a mad on that night. I'm sorry." And then he's sweet again.'

'Did you ever consider that a person's moods can change?'

'Mine don't. They didn't. Not when I was well.'

'Then you've held yourself under very strict control. I think you're aware of that in the light of what's happened to you. No one can go on day after day, always feeling pleasant inside. There has to be an ebb and flow.'

I sighed. 'I guess you're right.'

'Have you and Jay had many fights?'

'Oh, no. We never quarrelled. We never said mean things. We had a wonderful relationship.'

'How long have you been married?'

'Five years. Why?' Blood rushed to my face. 'What's wrong with being married five years without a fight? My parents don't fight. They've been married thirty-two years. I never heard them yell or curse or say rotten things to each other. . . .'

. . . 'Judy . . . listen to this.' Her face was beaming. 'Harold comes home from school today. He walked home with a little friend. You know, that Tommy, from up the block. The father's a plumber. So anyway, he comes in and he asks me, "Mommy, why doesn't Daddy throw a chair at you like Tommy's daddy does to Tommy's mommy?" How do you like that? A child's eyes . . . he wants to know why . . . Anyway, I ask him and he says they were saying loud words and then the fighting started. See how it is in some families? Judith, you're thirteen years old. Did you ever hear a shut up between Daddy and me? Or a go-to-hell? Did you? Did you?'

He had tilted far back in his chair and his fingers were curled under his belt. He was watching me with slightly closed eyes. I felt hot and chilly at the same time.

'What are you thinking about?' I asked, hesitantly.

Is this right? Should a patient ever ask the doctor what he's thinking?

'Well, it looks as though your environment set up certain standards for you. You never saw real anger or hostility. It's possible you grew up thinking it's wrong to show your own hostility or have others vent their anger on you.'

'You mean Jay?'

'Yes. And your boss. And your fear of having people criticize or make cutting remarks. And the shock of failing one exam can fit into this picture, too. Even myself.'

'You?'

'Yes. You always ask if I'm angry with you. Suppose I were. How would you feel?'

'Lousy. Hurt and lousy. I'd feel that you don't want me for a patient any more.'

His eyes were slightly slitted again. 'You're extending one incident of displeasure into an entire relationship.'

'And that's wrong?'

'Not wrong. But not healthy. Now what about that schoolmate of yours?'

'Oh, yes. I forgot. We've digressed so much. Does this happen with your other patients?'

'Quite often. Sometimes the digression is much more fruitful than the main topic.' He chuckled softly.

'Phyllis was always ahead of me. If I got 94 in Arithmetic she got 96. In the gym races she always ran a little faster. She always did things a little better than I could. I hated her. You know, I don't think I'll ever forget her. If I could draw I could sketch her for you. She was dark. Very dark. Sort of Latin looking. She had brown curly hair. Her eyes were green. Against her brown skin they made her look like a cat. Isn't it funny? Why should I remember her so well?'

'Was she the only competition you had in school?'

'No. There were other good students. But she . . . there was a wiriness about her. Tight. Like a coiled spring. We were friendly in a coolish way. Not close, but friendly.' I sniffed a laugh. 'I wonder if she knew of the rivalry between us.'

'Did she look like anyone you knew?'

'No. No one. Why? What would that mean?'

'I don't know right now.'

Again I flushed and shivered.

This conversation . . . there must be something . . . Phyllis a rivalry . . . his question . . . does she resemble anyone I know . . . maybe he sees something . . . some connection . . . won't tell me . . . or can't tell me . . . and I just can't seem to dredge it up. . . .

'Do you like cats?'

'Huh? Oh. Cats? No. I'm afraid of them. You never know what they're thinking. Whether they like you or not. When a dog's going to bite you can hear it and see it. He growls. His lips curl. You know. But a cat just sits and stares at you and then the claws come out. I told you Phyllis looked like a cat, didn't I? Well, that ties in, huh? But where? I mean, what does it prove?'

'Nothing, right now.'

'Do you see anything in it?'

'I don't know.'

He's honest. Admits when he's stumped. But do I like this honesty in him? Do I want him to be human or superhuman? Demi-god doctor or plain man?

I looked at my watch. The session was over.

'Time's up, huh?'

'Just about.'

'It's funny. Today I didn't talk about Gary at all.'

'Do you feel we should have?'

'Yes. That's what I'm here for. That's my main problem.'

'Let's say it's the most pressing one. Certainly not the main one.'

'Well, I—oh, gosh! This is the second time we forgot about my father. I mean, the incident I wanted to talk about.'

'We'll start off with it next time. Will next Thursday be all right?'

'Yes. Sure.'

I wrote down the date in my notebook.

Two hours with me and he gets almost as much as I make in a week. Can't stop thinking how much this is costing. That's bad. He's helping. Must remember that . . . and all the other things . . . get so

*tensed up as I leave him . . . can't wait to get it down in the diary.
Then I know I've really got it . . . that I won't forget . . . wonder
what he'll do when I leave? Thumb through a book to check on relationship between cats and compulsives? . . . And that stuff about my
parents. All that sweetness and light. And me, so scared of bitterness
and fights . . . scared of people . . . of my baby . . . scared to possess . . .
scared of everything . . . must have been born scared and haven't stopped
running . . .*

'I'll run along now, Doctor Borman. G'night.'

'Good night, Judith.'

''Bye' . . . I closed the door.

The trip home was a strange one. I manœuvred through the
crowded streets without any consciousness of having done it.
All my senses were turned inwards, trying to explore the path-
ways of thought the session had provoked. I was stunned and
awed. My God, I thought, there's so much to it . . . so much to
plumb and sound and weave together. It's exciting, almost, to
realize how much of me lives far below. Like an iceberg. No.
More like a volcano. I've blown up once from the fires inside.
What will this therapy do to me? Put them out? Expose them?
Control them? Make me know myself so that I'll be a different
person who still won't know herself? It's scary . . .

Thursday, March 8

'Hello, Doctor Borman.'

'Hi. (*Such a casual way he says hello. Feel like answering, Hi ya,
pal, what's new? Jay always greeted me with a Hi whenever I'd meet
him. Too offhand. Too cool for a wife. With Borman it's sort of cute.
It doesn't fit with the way he looks.*) How have you been?'

'O.K. But I get so nervous every appointment day. I start to
watch the clock in the office as soon as I get in. By the time I
come here I'm very tense. My neck hurts and my eyes burn.
You know, my eyes are terrible lately, I think I need my glasses
changed. I can't see the street signs well, or the cards on the
buses. There's always a pressure, and a blurriness. I don't
know, maybe it's tension.'

'How long have you worn glasses?'

'Since I was eight.' I leaned back in the chair and pressed my
fingers on my eyelids. 'What I could do with a month of sleep!

A week. Even eight solid hours. (*Whining to him. Always verbalizing my discomforts. Looking for sympathy. But he just sits there waiting for me to run out of complaints. Only ones who pay attention are Mother and Dad. Dad——*) Doctor Borman, I want to tell you about my father. He came in for the week-end again. Week-end! He gets here eight-thirty Saturday night and takes a ten o'clock bus back to New York Sunday night. Twenty-six hours. Big week-end. Anyway——'

'He lives in New York?'

'Yes. Didn't you know? My parents live in the Bronx. My father works every day. He's a salesman in an appliance store. Part of a chain. He's been there for thirty-two years . . .'

'*Judith! Daddy's home!' Loud. Strong. Then, a whisper. 'Ssh . . . he doesn't look so happy, I thought maybe he'd enjoy the testimonial dinner. But I know him. He probably sat there all night thinking of the twenty-five Christmases he spent a nervous wreck. And all the gall he's taken. From Jennings. The kicks in the pants. They started together. Did you know that? Sure. So now Jennings is a millionaire president. It hurts to think. If the old man were alive today . . . the first president . . . things would be different. He always liked Daddy, the old man. He used to keep in touch with the men. But Jennings . . . a gansa macha now . . . a big shot . . . a home in Long Island . . . anyway, as soon as we see Harold out of college Daddy's going to give up being manager. Who needs it? The aggravation? The hours? All the headaches? Let him be a plain salesman and go home at six o'clock. . . . Look. Don't say anything when you see the watch. Daddy thinks it's cheap. He saw the one Goldberg got at last year's dinner'* . . .

She walked into the hall where he was hanging up his coat. '*Hello, honey. You hungry?*'

'*Nah. Maybe a cup of tea.*'

'*So how was it?' She spoke very casually.*

'*Like any dinner. Filet mignon. Mine was a little tough.*'

I stood in the doorway, trying to think of something to say that wouldn't disturb him. '*Any dancing girls, Daddy?*'

He frowned. '*What's the matter. You crazy? At a testimonial dinner?*'

'*For heaven's sake, I'm just joking!' I looked at Mother's eyes. They were veiled. I couldn't tell whether she was angry or not.*

'*So who spoke?' she asked.*

'*Jennings. And the editor from "Appliance News". The same malarky as last year.*'

It was impossible for me to keep still: '*Did you stand up when they called your name?*'

'*Sure I stood up. Jennings made a remark - how we both started together. That both of us are veterans. Veterans.*' His mouth moved as though he were tasting something bitter. '*So maybe he wanted me to show him my battle scars.*'

'*Do you have the watch, Dad?*'

'*Yes.*' He took out a thin brown box from his suit pocket and opened the cover. '*See?*' He turned the watch over. '*My name on the back. And the date.*'

'*It's beautiful*', I said.

'*Is it gold?*' Mother asked.

'*Of course it's gold*', I snapped. '*Isn't that silly? You think they'd give him a plated one?*'

'*You don't know Jordan Company.*'

I tried again. It hurt me to see them . . . so glum . . . so devoid of emotion. Why couldn't they laugh a little?

'*Well, Dad, does it seem as though twenty-five years have gone by?*'

He looked at me, then took off his glasses and blew on them and held them up to the light. He sighed. '*Ye-ep. Twenty-five years. To-night, when my back hurts and my knee hurts it feels like a lifetime. Ma . . . you going to make the tea?*' He put his hand on my shoulder. '*Yes, darling. Tonight I'm an honour member. Tomorrow morning I break my back and kiss their arse.*'

'He comes in every week-end to see her. I mean us. That's why I'm so anxious to get well and take over. So my mother can go home. He's all alone there. I feel so guilty. A grandmother should come to visit her daughter. Not live with her. Not have to leave her husband alone.'

'Are you ashamed?'

'No. The close family knows what happened. He tells strangers . . . people in the apartment house, that I'm working. I'm not ashamed. I'm just guilty tearing them apart this way.'

'Are they very attached to each other?'

'Terribly. Particularly my father. He's so dependent on her. You know, sometimes it annoys me. The way he's under her thumb. She rules him. He's afraid to express himself. He grovels. It makes my skin crawl.'

Suddenly it was difficult to talk. My throat was closing. I swallowed hard.

'Two weeks ago he came to see us. He was talking to me while he washed his hands for supper. He said something about Gary . . . how precious he was . . . and why can't I love him. I got excited and yelled. And right away she's there . . . like a mother shutting up a child who spoke out of turn. Why is he so afraid of her? Why doesn't he stand up to her?'

'Is that what you've wanted to do?'

'When?'

'When you were young?'

'Yes. I think so. I wanted him to be strong. To be a match for her. To fight back. Do you know, every time there's a decision to make . . . anything . . . whether to go for a walk or go to a film . . . he looks at her for the signal. I can't stand that. He never wins. She owns him. And he accepts it. And he comes back for more.'

'Maybe he's a very dependent sort of person.'

'Yes, he is. But he leans on her so much it's disgusting. Oh, I know that's a strong word. But he worships her and I can't stand it.'

'Why not?'

'I don't know. Say, are you hot? I'm so hot I'm sweating.'

'Do you want me to turn down the steam?'

'Don't bother. Well, yes. Would you?'

He got up and shut the steam valve on the radiator.

'See? I said "don't bother" automatically. I don't like to ask favours of people. Have them put themselves out for me. This time I was honest with you.'

He was back in the chair. 'How do you feel?'

'Very uncomfortable.'

'That's expected when you start breaking old habit patterns. Now. You were telling me about your father worshipping your mother.'

Very nervous. Sorry I started this.

'What was I saying?'

'You couldn't stand it. And I asked you why.'

'I don't know why. No. That's not true.' My fist crashed on the arm of the chair. 'He loves her so much and she doesn't return it. He goes to kiss her. She gives him her cheek. He tries to caress her. Pull her down on his lap. She wriggles away. Says she's ticklish. Or there's something on the stove. Always an excuse, so he can't love her. It used to be a standing joke round the house. I'd say, "Mother, I don't know how you and Daddy ever conceived children. You're always running away from him. He can't catch you." '

Doctor Borman smiled. 'Maybe your mother is self-conscious. Doesn't like to show affection in front of her children. Was she affectionate with you?'

'I don't remember clearly. We always kissed good night. And good-bye. Formal things. It's hard to remember . . . I . . . No. There *were* times . . . I would want to cuddle her . . . or get on her lap . . . I was young then . . . to touch her . . . she always put me off, sort of . . . now, wait. Maybe I'm wrong . . . I can't seem to remember it as a definite thing. It could be it was something I wanted to do . . . but never tried . . . I'm all mixed up. I'm sorry.'

'It looks as though you saw yourself in your father. Trying to get physical love from her. A constant reaching out and being rebuffed.'

His words were spoken low. But they boomed in my ears. 'Yes . . . yes . . .' I said.

This hurts. Until you want to cry . . . and cry. For shame . . . for love . . . for loneliness . . . for wanting . . . everything . . .

Tears clogged the back of my throat, salty-bitter and burning.

'Right now I could cry until you're washed out of here on a flood.'

'Why?'

'I don't know. But I'm not going to. It'll cost me money.' I sniffed. 'Time is money here. My time. Your money. Now I feel silly. Giggly. I want to say crazy things. Why?'

'To cover up your feelings?'

'I guess so. Yes. You're right. I've always done that. Escape on a laugh, you know? It's like running away.'

'Was your father affectionate with you?'

'Very.'

Veryandveryand muchmuchmuch.

I saw his face and body fill the room. He was all spread out, each part of him moving in slow disarticulation. Kissing lips, puckered to touch my cheek with wetness and sweetness. Nose nuzzling my neck, sniffing, searching. Small warm eyes reading my face. Hands reaching to pet and pat. Arms lifting me to a long-legged lap. Love leaking and spilling and flooding all over me. Drowning me. Choking me.

I coughed. 'You know. I can't understand it. He was so loving. He used to sniff my neck. Grab my hand and hold it next to his chest. Things like that. But I couldn't stand it. I don't know how it was when I was very young. But later on I never let him hold me on his lap. Funny! Even on dates I never liked to sit on a fellow's lap. I couldn't put my weight on him. It was very uncomfortable. I didn't like our bodies touching. Is there some connection there, do you think?'

'Go on.'

'About what? My father?'

'Yes.'

'That's all. I was always pulling away from him. Just like my mother, huh? I hated her for running from him and I did the same thing. I still do. I get so flushed when he bends to kiss me. It happened two weeks ago. I wanted to kiss him on the lips but I did just what Mother did. I turned my face.'

'How do you feel when he tries to fondle you?'

Why did he say 'fondle'? Sounds dirty.

'I feel very uncomfortable. Like a baby. A child. I want him to stop. But I can't tell him that. He wouldn't understand. And he'd probably forget and do it again. He's like a child himself, sometimes. He's so easily hurt. He's so good. He means well. I don't want to hurt him.'

'Why?'

'Why? Because I love him.'

'Is that all?'

'What else?' I was puzzled now. And frightened. Borman's face was quiet. He didn't sniff or touch his moustache. His eyes were rooted on me. His voice was soft and insistent.

'There is something else. I think you're afraid of your own positive feelings for your father.'

'W-what do you mean, positive?'

'Love feelings. Feelings of attraction.'

Sweat oozed from every pore of my body.

My God, he's trying to——

'Are you telling me I . . . I *want* my father? That's crazy. I mean, that's incest!'

'Why do you say incest?'

'Well, that's what you're implying, isn't it?'

'No. They are very normal feelings.'

'I'm normal if I'm in love with my father?'

'Yes. Every girl is, as a child. And every young boy wants his mother.'

'Is this . . . this idea . . . is it yours?'

'No. It's Freud's.'

Oh. Freud. Great God Freud.

'You're talking about the Œdipus complex, aren't you?'

'Basically, yes.'

'Œdipus was a man, wasn't he? A Greek? And the woman . . . I forgot her name.'

'Electra.'

'So that's me, huh? Well, I just can't accept it. You say it's normal. How can it be normal?'

'Because these are the feelings we all have as children.'

'But I'm grown up now.'

'Most of us make an adjustment as we grow older. It's not something we're aware of. We just come to accept the fact that we can't have the parent we favoured.'

'And I favoured my father?'

'Yes. His approach to you seems very spontaneous and persistent. In his way he's openly expressing his own need for affection. You've held back your feelings.'

'Suppose my mother were more loving, more outward? Would it have been different?'

'I don't know. Perhaps. But from the child's standpoint sometimes it's better for the favoured parent to be more detached. Your father is a seductive person. He can't control his physical affection for you. That can cause a lot of guilt.'

Seductive. He makes him sound like a woman. Slinky. Slimy. Sexy. That's not Daddy. Daddy's simple. Kittenish. Childish.

'Guilt in whom? I'm sorry, Doctor Borman. I know I sound stupid. But it's so hard to understand.'

'In yourself. Because he stirred up a lot of feeling in you. You couldn't respond because you thought it was wrong. Unconsciously, that is. This is something a child is never aware of.'

'So I ran away from him. Is that what you're saying?' I wiped my hands on a tissue. It was soaked with sweat.

'Yes. That business about not sitting on men's laps. That has a definite connection with your father. And now you're finding it hard to kiss him under ordinary circumstances.'

'Or touch him. You know, I'm afraid to touch him. When he gets close to me I . . . get so confused. No. Mixed up. No, that's not right.' I swallowed hard. 'I know the word but I don't want to say it.'

'What is the word?'

Allrightallrightallright. Might as well pick me clean.

'I get . . . excited. As if he were another man . . . a stranger. Or my husband. My husband's like a stranger now. There's very little sex with us lately. I'm not interested. I have no patience. I'm too tense. And the nights he's home he never approaches me. He goes to bed early. I stay up and talk to my mother. I hate to go to bed. I still don't sleep well. Then when it happens . . . sex, I mean . . . it's more like brushing your teeth. Going through the motions. Something you do because you have to do it. My father doesn't understand why I'm sick. He never will. But when he comes into the house . . . it's like . . . I'm home again . . . Home . . . you see?'

The word stuck in my throat. And my hands began to wring out tears. They flowed hot and wet. I couldn't stop them. I hung my head.

How many times has he seen tears like mine? Men and women who crumple and heave, their faces contorted, as they strip themselves of the mask of self-respect and weep for shame and guilt.

'I feel . . . that I want to go to him . . .' I fumbled for tissues and held them to my eyes. 'Be picked up. Bury my head. Cry. Like I'm crying now. But the moment he bends over me I run.'

My eyes were still averted as I waited for him to speak. He was so still I had to look at him. His face showed no sign that he had been a witness to an outburst. I blew my nose loudly.

'I hate to cry. It's so messy. And I get such a splitting headache. (*What the hell's with him? Is this a monologue? What does he want from me? Must I bang my head on the wall before I get a rise from him? But I have to know. I have to know.*) What . . . should I do? Accept the fact that I'm in love with my father?' My hands spread helplessly.

'Yes.'

'You say it so calmly. As if it were nothing. And it's so important.'

'How should I say it?'

Whisper. Lower your eyes. Don't sit there so blandly as though you're telling me I should look at the sun, it's shining.

'I don't know. It's not a pretty thing.'

Shocking. Disgusting. Ugly. Terrifying. That's what it is, don't you see?

'I want you to think about it. When you're not so upset. Then let me know how you feel next week.'

I checked my watch with his little clock.

'Yes. All right.'

He waited until I was in my coat. Then he stood up, the line of his body cutting into the yellow light from the overhead bulb.

'Next Friday? Same time?' I asked. I was too tired for the amenities of leave-taking.

'Yes. Same time.' His pale eyes washed over me.

As I turned to manoeuvre out of the narrow office door. I saw him standing there, tall and silent.

Are you my strength or my undoing? Do you force self-dissection to cure or confuse? Your questions are like knives. They hurt and hurt and hurt and——

The door closed. I stood in the hallway feeling fingers of exhaustion creep through my body.

Tired, so tired. Like after shock treatment. A shock. A jolt. Shock of knowing. Learning. Forced learning. Painful. Shameful. Won't believe. Can't believe. Is it the truth? IS IT?? Daddy, dear Daddy, come home to me now. Hello, Daddy? How are you? Have a good trip? Is it cold in New York? Bend down, Daddy . . . let me kiss you. Full on the lips. Mmm . . . your face is cold. Good to see you, Daddy. By the way, Daddy . . . a little bit of news. I'm in love with you, Daddy. Yes. Really I am. Not love. I said IN LOVE. Just found it out this week. The touch of you. The smell of you. The feel. Like man and woman. Daddy's girl loves Daddy.

'Jay?'

'Hhhmm?'

'Can I talk to you for a minute?'

'What is it?' He was reading in bed. The light from the wall lamp shone on his head.

'You're studying.'

'No. Not really.' He underlined a paragraph and then clicked in the lead on his pencil.

'You know, Doctor Borman is a good doctor. He's smart. He's making me see things even though they're unpleasant.'

'What things?' He turned the page.

If HE talked to ME, I'd stop reading. I'D listen.

'Can you listen and read at the same time?'

'Sure.' He smiled. 'In high school I did homework with the Make Believe Ballroom on the radio. Why? You think I'm not listening to you?'

'No. But I wanted to talk.'

He put the pencil in the binding and closed the book. 'Go ahead.'

I flushed. 'You sound so dramatic. As if you're threatening me.'

'Threaten? All I said was go ahead and talk.'

'You act like you're doing me a favour.'

'Look. You're the one who's dramatic. Everything's a production with you. What should I do? Stop breathing when you talk? The way your parents do?'

'Why bring my parents into this?'

'Because I feel like it.'

I looked at the closed bedroom door. Mother was reading two rooms away. If I yelled, she'd hear me. I forced my voice down.

'You know something? I don't think you care if I'm getting better or worse. You're so damn distant. And that blah look you give me. Those one-syllable answers. Yes. No. Go ahead. What is it? Why don't you talk?'

My fingers plucked at the blankets.

'I don't feel free to talk. Your mother is always around. I don't like it.'

'What should I do? Send her home?'

'No.' He sighed. 'You're not ready to be on your own yet.'

The blood rushed to my cheeks. 'Now what kind of a crack is that?'

'No crack. I'm just saying you're not ready to take over the responsibility of the house yet.'

'It happens to be true', I said, sarcastically. 'But how the hell do you know? You never ask me how I'm doing, or if I found out anything important.'

'Therapy's not a treasure hunt.'

'I know that, wise guy!' My teeth were gritted now. 'Oh, you think you're so smart. An inscrutable Sphinx. Sees all. Knows all. Says nothing.'

He looked at me and smiled. 'Quiet, everybody. The actress is on stage. Big scene.'

'Cut it out! Oh, it's no use. You avoid me when you can and when you can't you fight.'

'I fight? You're the one who always starts it.'

'Sure. Sure. It's all my fault. And my fault for getting sick, huh? It doesn't matter to you that I'm trying to get well . . . that I'm seeing a doctor . . . that I want to talk to you about myself and the baby . . . and other things . . . you just don't care.'

'I'm sorry you feel that way.'

'Sorry? You don't know how to be sorry. You're too busy being the Great Stone Face. Mister Unapproachable.'

'You love to exaggerate, don't you?'

'That's the way I feel. And Borman told me feelings are more important than facts. So there, smarty!'

'Do you enjoy tearing me down?'

'I'm crazy about it. I just love to fight like this.'

'You do.'

'I do *not!* I hate fights.'

He laughed. Suddenly and bitterly. 'That's the best joke I've heard all week.'

'I'm so glad I make you laugh.'

'I've got early rounds tomorrow. I'm going to sleep. Do you want this light?'

'No.'

He switched it off. Then I heard him turn over in bed.

I could kill him. If I had a knife I'd kill him. So goddam smug. So stony. So cold. Like a rock. If I killed him, could I reach him? Could I? Could I?

Friday, March 16

'It's worse than it ever was. It's awful.'

I sat in his chair with my hands plumped in my lap and an expression on my face that seemed to say, See? You've complicated things. You messed me up terribly and you're not going to get away with it. I'm throwing the whole thing back in *your* lap.

'What's worse?' There was a trace of a smile in his eyes.

'Everything—My parents and Jay—Last night we had a fight. I——'

'Let's take one thing at a time.'

'All right. About my parents. I'm squirming inside. With embarrassment. I watch them like a hawk. I'm suspicious of every remark, every word we say to each other, every gesture we make. When my father kisses me now I want to scream. And I feel so dirty. As though I've discovered an ugly secret about us.'

I lit a cigarette and drew hard on the smoke. It bit my lungs.

'What I'm trying to say ... this damn awareness you've given me. Now I know how Pandora felt when she opened the box and the snakes came out.'

He leaned back. His eyes were still amused.

'Awareness is the beginning of insight. And that can create anxiety, too. You have to live with it. Temporarily. Until you can develop new responses.'

'Well, I can't tell them, can I?'

'No. That wouldn't be wise.'

'Then what should I do?'

'What makes you think you have to do something?'

'But——'

'Just tolerating this new anxiety is enough.'

'I'm sorry. I don't understand.'

'You're going to re-experience these new feelings in many situations. Then you'll start to handle them spontaneously, without any conscious effort to change. You'll be more comfortable, more at ease with them.'

'Doctor Borman, now don't get angry. I mean, annoyed. I know I'm a nudje. I——'

He chuckled.

'I don't mean to press you for answers. I just can't help it. (*Press against you. What would it feel like? That long, lean body. So long. How is he in bed with his wife?*) Every time you use that word spontaneous I think to myself, what the hell does he mean? How can something come without a plan? You said that about the baby. That I'll grow to love him without forcing myself. But I still can't believe it.'

He picked up a pencil and twirled it between his fingers.

'I don't think I've ever done a spontaneous thing in my life. To tell you the truth, spontaneity scares me. It's like a sudden change. Only inside me. I have to have a reason for everything I do. Every way I feel.' I hurried on before he could reply. 'I know, I know. It's all part of being so compulsive. But you know how bad I am. So you ought to know that a person like me . . . is . . . well, they get scared of things without pattern. Without order. And that's what spontaneity means to me. Do you understand?'

'Yes.'

'And you still want me to ride . . . float . . . just hold it inside and not do anything about it?'

'That's right.'

I crossed my arms against my chest like a fishwife.

'I'll be dead before I'll learn to be spontaneous.'

He laughed. 'Let's see what happens. Let it ride, as you say.'

I shrugged. 'All right. But it's only because I believe in you. I mean, I think you're smart.'

'Do you want to tell me about Jay now?'

'Jay? Oh, you mean the fight? You're damn right I do. What the hell am I working for? For money. For you. To sleep at night? To love my baby? To understand my relations with my parents? What am I knocking myself out for if my marriage is shot?'

'Are you asking me or telling me?'

'I don't know. I feel lousy today. Depressed. Oh, not like before. I know what's wrong. It's Jay. The damn thing is there's no real issue. We're just drifting from each other. He's not interested in me any more. He's all inside himself. Never tells me what he's thinking. When I try to talk to him—believe me, I try—he shuts me out.'

'What do you mean?'

'Just that. He keeps on reading. He's always reading. He answers in monosyllables. And he sets his face in that tight, hard way I can't stand. Why does he do this? I'm trying to get better. What does he want from me? Is he punishing me? I tell you I hate him. He's so mean, so hard. He has no feelings. None at all.'

I had to take off my glasses and rub my fists in my eyes.

The sniffle and snuffle. The dabbing hankie. The blowing and choking. So embarrassing to cry. Yet he doesn't even look away. Just watches and waits until I get over it with his face empty of pity or censure. How long does it take for a man to look with dispassion on the grubby misery of others?

'I'm all right now', I sniffled. 'God, how I hate to cry in front of you. Doctor Borman, why doesn't he talk to me? I want to talk to him.'

'I don't know.'

'That's all right. I didn't think you would. You've never met him.'

I looked at my watch. 'Great. Ten minutes gone from the hour and nothing accomplished.'

'Do you feel you must accomplish something every time?'

'Yes. Aren't you supposed to?'

'No. You still think of this room as a classroom and of me as the instructor.'

'Right now I don't know what I think. I'm so mad . . . and sad . . . I——'

'You're evading your feelings.'

'Doctor Borman, I'm so full of feelings I could scream. My father . . . my mother . . . this thing with Jay——'

'Maybe that has something to do with it.'

'I don't understand.'

He played with the pencil again. 'Well, these past two sessions we've been discussing what I'd call potent material. And I think you're carrying these new feelings away from here and into your close relationships.'

'You mean that I'm so upset about my parents and me that I'm harping on him?'

'Something like that. Yes.'

'Well, it's not true. He shut up like a clam even before I started with you. He's a million miles away from me. Even if I wanted to fight I can't get to him.'

'Is that important?'

'Of course it's important! He's my husband, isn't he? We're supposed to be close. Especially now. I want to feel rapport with a person. I can't stand being snubbed, being shut out. It hurts. I'm very sensitive.'

'About what?'

'Everything. When I was young it was my looks. I knew I wasn't pretty.'

'Did anyone tell you that?'

'No . . . no . . . I just knew it.'

'I see.'

I'm lying. Can he see it on my face? Oh, hell. Might as well tell him . . .

'It's not true. Somebody did. I mean something happened once. I must have been nine or ten. I played with the kids around the block. Mostly with girls. Sometimes we'd join the boys. There was one fellow. He was a year or two older than I was. He was the leader of the boys. He didn't play actively. I think he had a weak heart. They called him the Professor. He always made up weird games. His name was Howard Wasserman. I'll never forget him. Real blond and pale, with a nose like Bob Hope, and a thin mouth, and his face was freckled. I don't know how it started. I didn't fight with him. But one day he called me a baboon. Ape face. And the next day another boy yelled out, "Yaah! Here comes the baboon." And soon they were all doing it. (*Funny. Sitting here telling him this. Twenty years ago and it feels as if it's happening now. This*

minute. Almost as though that little bastard were standing across the
room and calling me names.) I started to look in the mirror and
turn my face from side to side to see if I really looked like an
ape. I kept telling myself I must be ugly. Why would he use
that kind of a tease? But I still went downstairs after school.
I wouldn't give him the satisfaction of knowing that he had
hurt me. I made believe I didn't hear. But I heard it all right.'

'What happened?'

'Nothing. He moved away. Years later I met him. We talked
about college. He was going to Law School. I kept talking and
thinking, you goddam louse. You don't remember, do you,
how you hurt me? How could you be so mean? I hope you
drop dead.'

'Is that all?'

'That's all. But I still hate him and I still feel ugly every time
I think of it. You know, I think that whole thing increased my
inferiority complex.'

'Do you feel you have one?'

'Yes. About my looks. That I'm not pretty.'

'Were there any other incidents?'

'No. Not that I can remember. My father used to call me
monkey-face when I was real small. But he didn't mean anything by it. It was just his way of playing. He said a lot of
funny things.'

I moved my hand aimlessly, as if to scatter the words and
dilute their impact.

'Monkey-face? Did you think that was funny?' His eyes
narrowed.

'Yes. Look, it doesn't mean anything. I don't know why I
mentioned it.' My voice was edgy.

He said nothing.

What are you staring at? Those baggy eyes. Going to frame up
another trap question? Knew I shouldn't have started with this thing ...

'Doctor Borman, I know what you're thinking. That every
little thing I say is important. Even if I say it by accident. That
I'm trying to protect my father. Keep blame away from him.
Well, I——'

I was cutting the air with my fingers, waggling them at him
as a mother does when she lectures a child.

'I think you're . . . oh, what the hell! I'll tell the truth. It did bother me. Very much. I hated it when he called me monkey-face. But I couldn't tell him to stop. I loved him too much.'

I sighed and sat back. The tension drained away.

'A minute ago I hated you. I didn't want you asking questions about my father. I shield him, don't I? He's my favourite. Oh, God, this is hard work. Forcing out things I don't want to talk about. I work harder here than I do on the job with that bitch on my neck. How I hate her! Maybe I'm jealous of her, too. She's quite attractive. You know, maybe I hate everyone who's good-looking. Oh, when I think of the hours I spent staring in the mirror, trying to find the good side of my face. You're a man—you wouldn't know the things girls do when they're growing up. Well, I never found it. The pretty outside part. So I made the best of what I had.'

'What was that?'

'Brains and a good figure. I must have been fifteen or sixteen. I popped.' I laughed sharply. 'No. Not physically. Psychologically. My entire personality. I became a real wisecracker. Sharp. Fast. Always good for a laugh. Life of the party. I used to tell myself, mingle if it kills you. At parties I'd break into a circle of boys to swap a dirty joke or ask one of them to dance. I was a very good dancer. Are you listening to me?'

'Why do you ask that?'

'You look like Jay right now. Sort of glazed. I never know if he's really listening. You look like you're a million miles away.'

'I see. Well, I am listening. I don't have a very animate face. Does Jay?'

'No.'

'Tell me more about your adolescence. Those parties.'

'I just knocked myself out, that's all. I wanted to be wanted. I tried to attract men with everything except my face. The way I walked. And held my body. The provocative remarks. The jokes. They must have thought, oh, brother, what an easy mark for petting. They didn't know that all I wanted was a date. I used to keep a diary. On the back page I'd list every date I had for the year. The name of the fellow. Where we went. I'd spend hours comparing one year against the next.

If I was busy I'd think, men want me. They want me and like me. They're taking me out. Me. Funny-looking me.'

'Is that how you thought of yourself?'

'Yes. Another thing. I never felt pretty on the inside, either. I mean like a real woman. Delicate. Feminine. I was always more at ease in sports clothes. Slacks. I would put my hands in my pockets like a man and walk with long steps and hold a cigarette the way a man does. Like this.'

I rolled my cigarette between thumb and forefinger. I giggled.

'This is funny. I'm telling you how I liked to act like a man. But you know what I did when I was eighteen? I bought black mesh stockings. The kind chorus girls wear. Very sexy. I was meeting my friends to go to a dance and I'm standing alone on a subway station platform. All the men . . . eyed me up and down. I felt so peculiar. Cheap and excited and thrilled and embarrassed, all at once. I watched them watching me and I thought—funny how I remember this—I thought, makes no difference who you are. College boy or bum. With these black mesh stockings and a short tight dress I can attract you. I have power. Can make you look and made you want. I——'

Suddenly the memory soured.

'Doctor Borman, what was I? What am I? A male woman?' I tittered nervously. 'A freak?'

'We all have male and female characteristics. You seem to have adopted masculine traits because you felt you weren't pretty in a world where girls should be pretty.'

'But the way I acted? So trampish. So . . .'

'You were also trying to prove yourself as a woman. Physically, that is.' He slipped his hand between his crossed knees. 'But I think you've wanted to be a man all along.'

I took his words lightly. 'Oh, yes. If a girl isn't pretty she doesn't like being a girl. I can see that.'

'No. There's more to it than that.'

He flicked his eyes to the clock.

'The hour's up?' I asked.

'Almost.'

'Doctor Borman, I'm going to tell you something. And I bet there are other patients who feel the same way. I hate you when

you look at that clock. Oh, I know you have to. You can't give
me all day. But it's like a door slamming in my face. I feel so
shut out and shut up. Bang! Finished! You're through!
'Bye, 'bye.'

'How would you like me to end the session?'

'I don't know. Maybe a catapult. Something that lifts me
out of the seat and out of the door. No. I'm just joking. But
it's such a let-down feeling.'

'You mean *I* let you down?'

'Well . . . yes. The moment the hour is up. No matter what
we're talking about. You drop me like a hot potato. I feel
humiliated. Cut off. I want to hold you. I mean, hold your
attention. Make you forget the clock. But you don't. You never
do.'

His head bobbed slowly. 'I see. Tell me, what kind of people
want complete and constant attention?'

'I don't know.'

'What age group, would you say?'

'Children, I suppose. You think I'm acting like a child, is
that it?'

'Yes.'

'But I'm not the only one who feels like this. Aren't there
other patients who resent it the way I do?'

'Yes. There are others.'

'Then you should advertise yourself as a child psychiatrist.'

I tittered to conceal a rush of hostility. He didn't smile back.

'A person who's emotionally mature can accept a reality
situation without feeling rejected or humiliated. A child can't
distinguish his own demands from reality. He can't modify
his wants.'

I had gathered up my clothing. We were both standing now.

'So I've got a child's mind, huh?'

'No. I didn't say that. Emotions and intellect can be as far
apart as we are to the nearest star.'

'Then what should I do? Be happy the hour's up? Leave with
a smile?'

He moved to the door. Then he turned and slipped his hands
into his pockets.

'Don't force yourself to do anything unnatural. As long as

you're aware of your feelings, that's important. Awareness is the first thing. Change comes later.'

'Good night, Doctor Borman.'

'Good night, Judith.'

The lift button buzzed sharply in the stillness. All the offices on his floor were closed.

Myomy. Stayed late today. Nice of that fellow. Doctor what's his name, to chat with me so long. Fifteen dollars nice. Maybe I'll drop around next week. Just for the hell of it. To hear what else he has to say. Good place to kill an hour. Remember now. Just an hour. No more, no less. Oh stop it, for God's sake. Stop being so stupid-mad. He said important things. And you care what he says. Care so much it hurts. So get home, little girl. You are a little girl, you know? Get home. Head hurts. Body throbs. Eyes burn. Eyesight getting worse. Insight getting better.

Wednesday, March 21

'I'm so damned mixed up I don't whether I should get a bottle like a baby, wear skirts like a woman, or go to the bathroom standing up!'

He laughed. It was a hearty laugh. I was glad my joke had gone over. I had rehearsed it quite a few times, trying to express confusion with a funny crack.

'You promised to explain this man-woman business. Remember?'

'I didn't say I would tell you. Anything I tell you directly, without your participation, has very little value. I think you're aware of that, Judith.'

'Oh, yes, I am. But if you'd just explain a little bit. Help me over the blank spots. I'll think about it. I'll work on it. I really will. And I won't write it down. I've stopped keeping notes. I'm trying to let things jell by themselves, you know?'

He knows, all right. Knows I'm lying. But I don't care. If he'll just point to the roots, I'll dig them out.

I set my face in a mask of wide-eyed pleading and waited and watched his. He stroked his moustache with his thumb and pursed his lips slightly.

'You told me you're very uncomfortable with your father now?'

16

'Yes. I'm trying to accept it . . . the fact that I love him . . . but it's so hard. It's embarrassing. I keep saying I'm a big girl now. I should have been over this long ago. But I'm not.'

'I see. Any other feelings?'

'Isn't that enough? (*He's fishing for something. He's trying to help me. I've got to think . . . squeeze my brains until it comes out. . . . Like having a baby, that's what this therapy is.*) Uncomfortable. Embarrassed. Disgusted with myself . . .' I ticked off the words on my fingers and shook my head. 'That's all, I think. Oh, wait. I'm jealous, too . . . of my mother . . . for having him . . . I've told you this . . . her right to have him . . . she's his wife . . . I'm the daughter . . . the kid . . . who wants what somebody else has and can't get it. It's very frustrating. I'm mad. Mad at the whole damn mess. At myself . . . at Mother . . . everything.'

'Is that all?'

I snickered. 'Well, I sure as hell can't be mad at my father. It's not his fault. Oh, maybe a little . . . I watch him now and I see what you mean about him being seductive. But I'm not angry with him.'

'Most young girls are. Not consciously, of course. As I've pointed out, all these feelings are far below the conscious level. But subconsciously they want to hate the favoured parent when they see they can't have him.'

'But . . . but isn't a kid afraid that all the love will be taken away?'

'Well, in most cases the conflict is solved as the child grows up. He comes to accept the situation.'

'And that's it?' I spread my hands.

'No There has to be something else. A strong identification with the other parent. In your case, it would be your mother.'

'You mean if you want to be the kind of person your mother is . . . it takes the edge off the pain of not having your father?'

He nodded slowly. 'The girl wants to be womanly, and little by little she takes on a feminine role because it brings her closer to the mother.'

I frowned and rubbed my fingers across my forehead. 'But . . . my mother is domestic . . . she's womanly . . . she loves her

home . . . cooking, shopping . . . she's not restless or masculine
. . . she never wanted a career . . . she never complained about
raising children . . . why didn't I identify with her?'

'What do you think?'

'I don't know. Honest, I don't know. Oh, she had her faults.
Everyone does. She hovered. She worried too much and she
yelled a lot when she punished me. I was scared of her. I think
I'm still scared now. Sometimes I feel like I'm six years old.
I want to be at ease with her . . . But I'm not. I'm still afraid
I'll do something wrong and she'll yell and hit but of course
she won't because I'm grown. I know that, you see. But it's
there . . . it's still there . . . it's . . .'

My voice trailed off. I saw him bend to catch my words. I
saw his eyes, intent on my face. But there was something
sharper and clearer and more insistent in front of me, a sudden
coalescence of the nebulous into the real. I saw my mother and
myself. We were in the kitchen. She was washing dishes at the
sink and yelling at me for something I did. I watched her
rubbing, rinsing, scrubbing. I couldn't take my eyes from her
arms and hands. Because any minute . . . any minute now she'd
turn and grab me and I'd get hit. I got it before . . . an hour
ago . . . but it's not over. I can tell by her voice . . . I'm going
to get it again. I can't walk away. That'll make her madder . . .
so I have to stay and listen and I'm going to get it again. Her
hands . . . so strong and quick . . . so quick . . . you never
know when.

My voice came out husky and quivering.

'You . . . you can't get close to someone you're afraid of,
can you?'

'No.'

'But I loved her. She's my mother.'

I sat quietly.

'What are you thinking of?' he asked.

'I wanted my father. I couldn't have him. And I couldn't
hate him. I should have identified with my mother. But I was
frightened of her. I tried to grasp two things and ended up with
nothing. I've got a woman's body and I don't know who the
hell I am inside.'

'Whom do you think?'

'I don't know. More man, probably. Guess I've always wanted to be a man. If you can't lick 'em, join 'em.'

'Why do you say that?'

'Who knows?' I was flippant now. Tension was building again. I picked at a hangnail. It tore off and a drop of blood spurted out. I licked it away. 'You remember that song, "I Ain't Got Nobody". Well, I had a body, but no personality. So I manufactured one. I feel like a fraud. A stupid fraud.'

I waited for him to say something that would soothe or mollify. But he sat quietly and didn't speak. I became annoyed and had to drop my head so he wouldn't see the anger in my eyes.

These doctors! Nothing moves them to comfort or pity. They're never shocked, stunned, or sorry for you. The facts, ma'am, nothing but the facts.

His voice broke the silence. 'Why did you say "if you can't lick 'em, join 'em"?'

'Huh? Oh. I told you I don't know.'

'Are you sure?'

'No. I'm just so tired. And I'm "famished" enough as it is. Is it important that I analyse everything I say?' My voice was sacrcastic.

'It is, here.'

'You're right. I asked you to help me. I'm sorry. I'll try. But I really don't know. It just came out. You want me to think about it?'

'Yes.'

'Like free association?'

He nodded.

'O.K. If you can't lick them . . . you join them. If you can't beat them out . . . not beat, really. Win. Win something . . . I don't know. . . . Anyway, if you can't win from men, you try to be like them . . . I've told you this—I always wanted to be a man . . . be free . . . strong . . . walk big . . . move big . . . not mince like a woman. With a cackle and a giggle and a whisper——'

'Not all women do that.'

'I know. I'm exaggerating.' I sighed.

'What is it you want to win from men?'

'Is that what I said? I don't know. Just getting something.'

'Something material?'

'You mean money? No. I'm not a gold-digger. I was always a real cheap date. It's not money . . . it's their strength . . . their power . . .' My fingers clawed the air.

'Where is a man's strength, Judith?'

'Where? That's a silly question. He's strong because he's a man. He's got a man's body, a man's penis . . . a . . .'

My voice trailed away. I dropped my head and pressed my fingers against my cheeks. They were burning. I felt flushed all over. I struggled for words. None came. Silently I begged him to talk and to ease the pain of this sudden insight. But he sat there, not two feet away, and said nothing.

A shock, a shock, a damn dirty shock. How disgusting I am. How perverted. If I could swallow myself . . . crawl in a hole . . . can't look at him . . . I'll stare . . . I know I'll stare . . . the way I've done to all of them . . . without volition . . . not wanting to but having to . . . a lure . . . an ugly fascination . . . one by one as they walk by on the streets . . . or sit opposite on a bus . . . I try . . .

'Really, I try . . . I try to keep my eyes on their hats or their faces or count the buttons on their coats . . . but it's no good. Something pushes me to look at them . . . in that place . . . I don't know why. . . . It's almost as though I'm telling myself, checking, that's all, just checking. . . . But it wasn't checking. It was more like . . . like peeking. Dirty peeking. Looking at something you shouldn't.'

My fingers wrapped round the chair arms.

'I've been married for five years and I still have to stare. I'm seeing it but not believing it. Denying it . . . afraid of it . . . when we're in bed . . . and I caress him and run my hands along his body . . . every time I touch it I'm surprised. Isn't that crazy . . . surprised to find your husband has a penis and it's in the right place and it's big and hard? Sometimes I squeeze it and I get afraid. It's like holding something apart from his body. Something that grows and moves under my fingers . . . sensitive . . . so vital . . . so powerful. And I have to make jokes. I shake hands with it. I call it the little feller . . . I have to laugh at it. Or else I'll . . . I'll . . .'

'What?'

I pulled my hands back along the arms of the chair and pressed my elbows against the sides of my body, forcing air out of my lungs.

'Cry. Yeah. Cry. Or pull. Or squeeze too hard. Hurt him. Hurt him very much.'

Not his fault he's a man and he has it and I don't have it and I want it. Not his fault.

I looked at Doctor Borman now. The washed-out eyes were still open, still watching me with detachment. No flicker, no sparkle, no show of surprise. And now I thought thank God for him. For being a doctor. For harbouring no shame for me. I've said things to him I could never tell another. This tired, baggy stranger in a wrinkled suit. I don't even know his middle name or his home address or how many kids he has.

I smiled wanly. 'Now I know why psychiatrists never treat relatives or friends.'

'What do you mean?'

'If I knew you I couldn't say the things I've said. You understand?'

'Yes. I understand.'

'What the hell is wrong with me? Am I a sadist?'

'I don't think so.'

'Then what is this thing with me? . . . this obsession with the penis?'

'What do you think?'

'I want one. But it's not that alone. Not just physical.'

'A symbol of strength, perhaps?'

'Yes. Strength and power. The power of a man. But why do I envy them so much? Why do I want to hurt them?'

'I think it's a question of symbols again. A particular feeling about one person extended on to others.'

'One person? Which person? Who is it I want to hurt?'

'Suppose you try to tell me?'

'Jay. We're not getting along at all. I've told you how he is . . . so cold . . . so unfeeling . . . sometimes I want to hit him. It's Jay, isn't it?'

'Do you want it to be him?'

Shrewd, he is. Knows I'd like to hang this on Jay.

'Yes. I'm angry at him. But I don't think . . . I mean, I've felt like this for so long . . . this hunger . . . this envy . . . I can't remember when it started. Maybe I was born hating men.'

I tried to laugh, to break the strain and make him ease his probing. But his eyes refused to smile.

'All right. So I'm joking. But I honestly don't know. I was never raped or assaulted. You know, these shocking things girls experience and then they hate all men. I never had a father who beat me, who——'

Beat me. Did I say beat me? Before I said I want to beat men. Beat them, win them . . . a symbol, he says . . . can't remember when it started . . . must have been young . . . but Daddy didn't beat me . . . I loved him . . . I love him now . . . I . . .

'My father? It's my father?'

The words came out cracked and hoarse.

'It seems that way to me', he said.

I cleared my throat and sputtered. 'But . . . but . . . I thought you said . . . today . . . at the beginning . . . that I couldn't hate him . . . wanting him so much.'

'I said a child is afraid to hate the favoured parent.'

'Scared to hate the one she loves. Right? Right? This feeling . . . being let down . . . I couldn't have him . . .' I picked at the bloody fingernail again. 'I still can't . . . And I'm still mad, huh? No. Don't answer. I see. I think I see. When you're mad you want to hit back . . . But you can't hit your father, can you? You'll lose everything. Even the little bits of love you know are just for you.'

'Exactly.'

'So I tried to get at him through all the others?'

'Something like that.'

'But I still don't understand why I aped men. Liked to be masculine.'

'In a situation like yours there's a lot of conflicting emotions.'

'I see. (*See? Daughter. Daughter mad at Daddy 'cause Daddy's not for her. But don't tell Daddy. Don't tell anyone. Just take the hate and move it. Like a bundle of shit. And let it drop on everyone with a zipper on his trousers. Hate. Emasculate. And emulate. Want to be what you want to destroy.*) This is great. The more I find out about myself the worse it gets.'

'Worse?'

'Harder. It's not a pretty picture, you know. Not pretty at all. What a mess I am. Do you know anyone more "famished"?'

I looked to his eyes, not expecting an answer, but hoping for one. And then I saw the wards at State Hospital. And I remembered something Mother had said long ago, quoting an old Jewish parable: 'I wept because I had no shoes. Then I met a man who had no feet.'

Tuesday, March 27

He must have felt my cheeks burning through the telephone wires. I was terribly embarrassed to call him up like that. Perhaps there was someone in the office. Or someone lying on the couch. But maybe he was used to patients calling. And maybe some of them would barge into the office . . . if I had the guts that's what I'd do. I felt so lousy.

'Doctor Borman? Judith Kruger. I'm really sorry to bother you. Do you have a minute? I just had to talk to you. I'm sick again.'

'I can't hear you. Could you talk louder?'

'I said I'm sick again. Nervous. I'm shaking all over. I'm so scared. I don't know what's wrong.'

'Did something happen over the week-end?'

'Nothing, nothing. I didn't go anywhere.'

'Did you quarrel with Jay?'

'No, Doctor Borman', I croaked. 'Could I see you before Friday? Please?'

'I don't think so, Judith. I'm all booked up. Unless I have a cancellation. (*Really doesn't care. If he cared he'd make room for me, time for me. Maybe I'll cancel, too. I'll drop dead.*) Can you hold out until I see you?'

'I . . . I don't know. I stayed home from work today.'

'Do you want another shock treatment?'

'W-what do you mean?'

'I'm due at the Municipal Hospital tomorrow morning. Eight-thirty. At the out-patient clinic. I give shock therapy there. If you could get someone to go with you——'

He must be joking. If he thinks I'll let them do that to me. Again. He's trying to scare me, get rid of me. Knows I hate shock.

'No. I couldn't make it. Jay can't. And the baby. My mother . . . No. I'll be all right. I'll hold out.'

'If you want to call me up tomorrow, I'll be here from nine-thirty on.'

'Thanks.'

For nothing. . . .

'Try to keep busy around the house. Get your mind off the current anxiety.'

'All right. I'll try. Good-bye.'

Not to scream. Or dig fingers in flesh. Or bang walls with my head. Sure, I'll try. Be damned if I'll take shock again!

Friday, March 30

'Well! How are you? You didn't call, so——'

'I didn't have to! Doctor Borman, I'm so excited. I——'

'Why don't you sit down?' He smiled.

'Oh, yes. Sure.' I sat and then had to get up again. I wriggled out of my coat and threw it on the couch. 'I think I know what happened. What made me so upset. And I feel so good about it. I mean, being able to ferret things out for myself. (*Power. Power of self-discovery. Unassisted mind-fingers groping from why to why to still another yes, but why. Slowly pulling away the curtain of fear.*) Remember you asked me if anything happened? If I had a fight with Jay? I said no. And I wasn't lying. We just had a long talk. No arguments. We talked about the future. He asked me how I was doing with you. I said I'm making progress. I guess I sounded enthusiastic. And then he says, "I think I'll reapply for that residency from the University. This is the end of March. Maybe by July you'll be well enough to move. Your mother could come down with you for a few weeks to help you get settled. Or I could go down first and rent an apartment."

'He talked on like that. I answered him. I nodded yes. I mumbled maybe, let's see. And all the time I felt as though I were smothering. Choking. I got all knotted inside. And I didn't have the guts to say no. Tell him not to push me. That I won't be that well by July. And if he sets a deadline for me I'll never be ready. It was like somebody threw me on a merry-go-round. Every compulsive fear came back. I thought of moving and packing and travelling with Gary. . . . But the damn irony

of it was that I didn't realize what was happening. He finished
by saying he'll reapply anyway and we'll see. That we don't
have to go if I wasn't up to it. He kissed me good night and
that was that.

'The next day at work I started to shake. Every part of me.
All of a sudden. It got worse and worse. By the time I called
you I was in a terrible state. You know, the worst thing about
fear is not knowing why you're scared. And I remembered
how I was in the hospital. I think the memory of how I was
before and was it happening again made me more upset.
And then you asked if I wanted another shock. Doctor Borman,
you don't know what that did to me! I became even more
frightened because you thought I was sick. Sick enough for
more shock.

'When Jay walked in at the door that night I wanted to run
from him and hide. He saw how nervous I was. I told him I'd
called you. He asked me why. And I started to yell. I said,
"Because I felt like it. What did you want me to do? Check with
you first? I can't talk freely when I call the hospital. You're
always thinking the operator is listening. And if I cry it's no
good. If I make a scene I annoy you. You're tired of me
being sick."

'And I ran into the bedroom and slammed the door. I lay on
the bed and cried. When I stopped crying all I could feel was
hate. Like a fire in me. Then it cooled. And I started to think.
I forced myself to ask all kinds of questions. Why the outburst?
Why do I hate him now? So suddenly. Without a quarrel.
Why did the sight of him walking in at the door aggravate me?
I was actually afraid of him. His face. His voice. If he'd have
opened the bedroom door I would have screamed. (*Don't come
near me. Or touch me. Or pull me close to you . . . don't pull me . . .
don't want to go to you . . . go with you. . . . Don't make me move from
this bed . . . safe . . . big and flat and steady . . . slow and steady wins
the race . . . race against time . . . time running . . . running out . . .
who changed the time? . . . why am I running? run till you drop . . .
dead . . . dead . . . deadline . . .*) This cliché about a bolt of light-
ning hitting you . . . well, that's what happened. A welter of
thoughts . . . crazy thoughts . . . and then this one sharp
awareness. He wants me to be well by the summer so we can go

back South. I'm not ready to be on my own. I know it. But I'm afraid of disappointing him. That I'll make him angry. But I'm more afraid of moving and getting sick again.

'That's what was in the back of my mind since Saturday night. It took me two days of minor hell to make that simple connection. And the moment I realized it I felt better. It's like stumbling in the dark. Half-crazy with fear. Then a door opens. And I see things. And I understand them. Oh, the problem's still there. He wants me to go and I know I can't do it. But to see it. Like this. It's good. But why does insight come so hard?'

He held out a bony hand and contemplated it, smiling slightly.

'If I had a ready answer for that . . . All I can tell you is that anxiety is a means of escaping an unpleasant situation or emotion. I think you're aware of that by now.'

'Yes. I don't want to go back there. And I hate deadlines. Even little ones. Like getting to work on time. Or making supper. I get so nervous. I take everything so damn seriously. I'm afraid to fail.'

'You think you'll fail to meet this new challenge?'

'I know I will. I'm facing the facts and he isn't. He's pushing me. I don't want to be pushed.'

'That fear you spoke of. Fear of Jay touching you. Was that all you felt?'

'I don't understand.'

'I think it was more anger than fear.'

'No matter what I start to talk about it always ends up with me hating somebody.'

'You have a right to your feelings.'

'But I still feel guilty. And I can't go through life telling people off. People don't want honesty. If I told the truth all the time I wouldn't have friends. I couldn't hold a job. I——'

'You're skirting the issue. I said you have a right to your feelings. That doesn't mean flouting social codes with strangers.'

'How can I tell Jay I'm angry with him?'

'Just tell him.'

'I can't.'

'Why?'

I didn't answer. He leaned back in his chair. My nails scratched the chair arm. He watched me, his eyes neither bored nor impatient.

'I . . . I'm afraid he'll . . . this is so hard to say . . . he'll hate me too . . . he'll take his love away . . . if there's anything left of it by now . . . these past few months . . . the fights . . . so far from each other . . . I hate him for the way he treats me. But I love him.'

He didn't answer. The little clock ticked off the silence.

'Doctor Borman, sometimes you're like a Sphinx.' I giggled nervously. 'I feel creepy when it's so quiet. It's . . . it's embarrassing.'

'Why?'

Nothing to do. Just stare at each other. Stare and aware. Close. Too close. As if we were naked.

'I don't like another person watching me without saying anything. Jay does that lots of times. It makes me nervous. As though I've done something wrong. The silence shuts me out. You know, it's funny. One of the things that first attracted me to him was his quietness. His entire manner. So strong within himself. I used to think of him as my pillar of strength. Yeah, it's funny. Now that I need him I hate him because he doesn't talk.'

'He told you his ideas about going back South and——'

'And look what happened!' I broke in, heatedly. 'Of all the things to pick on.'

'He has to think of the future.'

'I know that. But it's other things. If I don't come to him . . . if I don't tell him how I'm doing with you or how I feel he never asks. *I'm* the one who's always pushing, pushing to get close . . . to open him up. It makes me so mad.'

'And you can't tell him you're angry?'

'No. I told you. I'm afraid of him.'

'Of losing his love. Is that what you said?'

'Yes. I think so. I'm not sure now how the hell I feel.' I slumped in the chair. 'When I came in here I was all excited. I'd worked through something by myself. Now it doesn't seem to matter much.'

I bolted up and shook my finger at him. 'Doctor Borman, do

you know that every time I think of our relationship now . . .
not you . . . I mean Jay . . . I feel like crying? Or . . . or . . .'

Hit. With fists. Smash him. His face. Crack it. Make it move.

'Or what?'

'Nothing. Why am I so afraid of him?'

'You answered that yourself. You think he'll take his love
away.'

'Yes. But . . . I feel . . . maybe there's more.'

'There is. And that's something I'd like you to think about.
On your own.'

'Why?'

'Well, you're making progress. You're gaining insight. But
you're always pressing me for answers. I'd like to see you work
through a situation on your own.'

'But I——'

'Now this isn't a homework assignment.' He smiled
crookedly. 'I don't want you to bring me any notes.'

'It's very hard for me to think without a pencil in my hand.'

'Then try to break the habit. All this writing down. It can
isolate you from your feelings about a problem.'

'Suppose I can't think of anything?'

'That's all right, too. I'm not challenging you to produce.
I'm not testing you. I just want you to dwell on your feelings
for Jay.'

'All right. I'll try. You know, until this thing happened with
him . . . about going back South . . . everything was sort of
quiet. I mean, we had no fights. I guess I was too busy thinking
about last time. God, I felt so creepy! So freakish. As though I
suddenly found out I had two heads. I wanted to run home and
take a bath. Get the dirt off. But it's not dirt, is it? It's what I
am and why I am and I have to understand it. But it's damn
hard, I'll tell you that. Damn hard. And I still stare at men.'

He chuckled. 'I didn't expect you to change in a week.'

'But now I know why I stare. Big improvement, huh?'

'Yes. I think it is. (*Another snake out of the box. Real ugly one.
But now I put it aside 'cause he wants me to work on Jay. That's bound
to be messy too. Everything's messy here. The more you dig, the——*)
There's something we didn't touch on in our discussion last
time. I'd like you to tell me about your brother.'

'Huh? My brother? Why?'

'What are your feelings for him?'

'I still don't understand. Harold. Of all people!'

'What's so strange about him?'

'Nothing. Nothing at all. It's just that he doesn't fit in the picture. I mean, in all the time I've been sick I don't think I've thought of him twice.'

'I'd still like to hear about him.'

'All right. (*Might as well humour him.*) Harold is an architect. He's four years younger than I am. He lives here in Philadelphia. I hardly remember him those weeks we lived in that Philly apartment. Mother told me he was a big help when they had to move to the new place. I was in the first hospital then. We see him about once a week. Sometimes less. He's tall. He wears glasses. And that's all.'

'What are your feelings towards him?'

'Feelings? He's my brother. What are you driving at?'

'You seem to be very reticent.'

'I'm not reticent. There's just nothing to say.'

'Suppose you let me be the judge of that.'

'O.K. O.K. You want to know my feelings for him. Well, I don't have many. I mean we're not very close. I don't care about him one way or the other. And that's how I felt from the beginning.'

'Beginning?'

'When he was born. You know how kids are supposed to be jealous when a new baby comes. Well, I wasn't. I was too busy playing with my friends. I never thought about him.'

'Are you sure?'

'Yes, I'm sure. I'll tell you something. I had a friend Anna. She was two years older than I was. She came in one day and saw him in his cot. And she said, "Oh, Judy, if I had a baby brother like that I'd love him so much." And you know what I said, "Come on, Anna. Let's play ball." And I pulled her out of the room.'

'You pulled her?'

'Oh, not really. I just wasn't interested in Harold when he was a baby. I never hit him. I never played with him. I just didn't bother. And I never felt jealous.'

'You're very sure of that?'

'Of course. I told you I never hit him. I——'

'Children can be jealous and not show it at all. Their jealousy can take many different forms. Indifference, for one.'

'But aren't kids' emotions all on the surface?'

'To a large extent, yes. But not always. I'm sure you're aware of that by now. Fear of punishment is a great deterrent.'

'You mean I was afraid to be jealous of him?'

'Let's say you were afraid to show it.'

'But I tell you I didn't care . . . I . . . (*Remember . . . remember . . . his words . . . long ago . . . first or second time you saw him . . . compulsions . . . steam from the kettle of self . . . can't show hate . . . can't show fear . . . have to let it out on toys and strings and little things . . .*) I was scared of my mother? That she'd hurt me if I hurt him?'

'Perhaps. But I think it was mostly fear of your own feelings about him.'

'So I played a game? I made believe I didn't care.'

He nodded.

I twisted my wedding ring.

'Funny . . . I was always so proud of myself. Proud that I never hurt my little brother. It made me feel different. Better than other people. But you're right. It sure came out later.'

'What do you mean?'

'I wasn't truthful before. I had lots of feelings for him. I hated his guts! God, did I pick on him! I was four years older and I used to win all the fights. Until he was ten or so. Then he learned a rabbit punch. You know that? You hit somebody with your knuckles right in the muscle of the arm. So I didn't hit him any more. I used my mouth. I teased him.'

'About what?'

'I don't know. I can't remember. No. There was something. I used to make fun of him. The way he was growing up. It . . . it sort of frightened me . . . his feet . . . his hands . . . his whole body getting bigger and stronger. Especially his hands. Harold liked to build things. He'd sit at a beat-up desk and play with the transformer from his old electric trains . . . or he'd make lead soldiers from a melting kit my uncle gave him . . . I'd watch his hands. See them growing large and square. Getting bigger every day. And I'd hate those hands. And I teased him. What was wrong with me?'

'What do you think?'

'I don't know. I just know I didn't like to see him getting ·bigger. It gave me the creeps to see him growing up.'

'Were you afraid he could hit harder now?'

'A little bit. But . . . it was something else. . . .' My hands curled into fists with the effort of thought. 'Almost as if he had no right to grow . . . to be stronger than me . . . have power . . .'

Where? . . . When? . . . you said that before . . . hating strength and power . . . big feet . . . big hands . . . and the thing between the legs. The sign . . . the symbol . . . the mark . . . of a man . . .

My voice was hoarse.

'He was my brother . . . and soon he'd be a man. I didn't want that . . . didn't like that . . . didn't want to see him strong . . . like the others . . . like all the others . . .'

I dug for a cigarette. The cellophane crackled. Then I made a pretence of looking for my matches. I had to keep busy.

There's a smug, didn't-I-tell-you-so look in his eyes and I don't want to see it. There has to be. He's so damn right. How the hell did he know about Harold? Neat little piece in the puzzle. Ten minutes ago I was laughing. Not important. Happens to be my brother, that's all. No meaning for me. No connection.

I forced a weak little smile and looked up at him. His eyes were quiet and calm.

'Every time I find something out . . . realize things . . . I always think you're smiling to yourself.'

'In what way?'

'Smug. Cocky. You sit there and watch me struggle . . . make me do it . . . and when it's over you're always right.'

'Do I look cocky to you?'

'No. It's not you. It's me. I . . . I have to learn you're not my torturer . . . that you don't get pleasure in proving me wrong . . . and I was wrong . . . not wrong, really . . . blind.'

'We see only what we want to see. And we allow ourselves to feel only the surface of our emotions. Those that give us the least pain.'

'If I had a sister instead of a brother, would it have been any different?'

'I don't know.'

'Poor Harold. I hated him double. For being born and for being a boy. I couldn't take it out on my father but I sure made up for that with him. Anyway, my teasing didn't stunt his growth. He's five feet eleven and weighs about one eighty. Doctor Borman, you don't know how my mother worried over him when he was little. She'd peek out of the window and compare him with his friends down in the street. ('*Look! Judith, look. That Arnie is almost two inches taller than Harold and they're the same age. And you see the other one? Look how fat he is. Harold is a peanut next to him. He's so skinny. He doesn't eat enough . . . does he eat enough? . . .*') She watched him like a hawk. And schtup, schtup, all day long. Green vegetable, yellow vegetable, cooked fruit, fresh fruit . . . she was a bug on proper diet. . . . He ate very well. I'll never forget. Every evening, he'd start his supper with whole wheat raisin bread and butter—this high—and then peanut butter on top of that . . . it came to here! And two slices of that, mind you. And she worried that he didn't eat. I used to laugh. But it bothered me.'

'What did?'

'I don't know. This whole eating business. Food, food, food. It was always on her mind. To have enough. When she shopped on Saturdays the orders kept coming from the stores until eight o'clock at night. She had cans of juices piled next to the refrigerator and they went almost to the ceiling. It bothered me. It still does. Maybe because I'm almost like her. When I shop I'm like a squirrel. I hoard. I'm always afraid I won't have enough or I'll run out of things. But she's worse. And now when Harold calls and says he's coming for supper she's like a dynamo. She gets a steak. Then she goes out and gets liver. Just in case. And she buys rye bread *and* pumpernickel *and* rolls. She asks if I have enough butter and I say yes but at the last minute she runs out for another half a pound.

'I get the feeling she doesn't think her son is coming, but some sort of giant maw. A creature with nothing but a mouth. And she has to fill it and fill it until it closes. Then she can relax and ask him questions and talk to him like a person again.'

'I see.'

He chuckled and his moustache twitched.

17

'It's funny to you?'

'Yes. You have a knack for vivid description.'

I flushed with an inner pride. Then I said, 'Well, I don't think it's funny. I hate her when she does that. Hovers over him. Caters to him. Puts so much damn food on the table.'

'Does he eat it all?'

'Yes. But that's not the point. It makes me angry to see her please him . . . that way . . . with food . . . like bribing . . . like buying love . . .' I held up my hand in anticipation of his comment. 'I know. I'm still jealous of him. But it's more than that. I watch her as she cooks and tastes and serves the food. ('*More sour cream, Harold? I didn't give you cucumbers because I know you don't like cucumbers but if you want cucumbers . . . Is the steak good? I mean, really good? . . . more salt, Harold? . . . Wait! I got green peas too. The little ones . . . the ones you like.*') She's like a servant to him . . . so nervous . . . so fearful there'll be something in the meal he won't like or he will like and want more and there isn't any more . . . it's as if their entire relationship depends on her success at the stove. I watch her and I'm ashamed.'

'Why?'

'Because I look at her and see myself. The way I am with Jay. It's like a disease. I caught it from her. Nervous supper-itis. I do the same damn things as she does. I watch Jay like a hawk when he eats the food I've cooked. If he stops in the middle I worry that he doesn't like it. If he doesn't ask for more I know he doesn't like it. And it's not him. Jay's not a fusspot. He's not a picky eater. It's me. Momma's daughter. Momma worries. So does daughter. Momma wants approval. So do I. And we work so hard to fill their bellies and feed their faces so we can get their love. Sometimes I stare at the meat frying in the pan and think, that's me cooking. In a minute I'll be on his plate. I hope I taste good to him; that he likes me; and says thank you. Then I'm safe. Until the next meal. And the next. There's no end to these offerings for love.'

Sunday, April 1

'Where do you want to go?'

'Anywhere. I don't care.'

He signalled left, cut into the line of cars merging at the circle and then veered right on to the highway.

'I remember this road. You went up to see me this way, didn't you?'

'Yes.'

That was when you loved me. When you cared. I was hospital sick. You travelled miles to spend two hours with me. To whisper in my ear that I'm your darling and I'm going to get well and it will take time. Nine months so far. Now I stick in your craw, don't I? Not sick. Not well. An unpredictable nuisance. A drag. I told Borman I'm afraid to lose your love. But I think it's gone already.

'The trees are budding already', he said.

'Yes.' I glanced out of the window.

'Enjoying the ride, sweetie?'

Sweetie?

'Oh yes, my dear darling.'

A tight smile came on his lips. 'What's the matter? Don't you want me to call you sweetie? I thought you like affectionate words.'

I stared at his profile. A ball of hate flew up to my throat and exploded.

'Who the hell do you think you're kidding? We've done nothing but fight for weeks. When I want to talk you cut me dead. You're so goddam into yourself and away from me. And now you call me sweetie. I'm not stupid. I feel things and sense things. You hate me because I'm still sick. Well, let me tell you this. I can't go back this July. Even if you decide to take the residency. I'm not ready and I don't want to move again and I don't want to leave Doctor Borman and I don't want to relapse. You don't know what I'm going through. Trying to keep myself under control. Trying to——'

'Now you listen to me a minute! Just because I don't jabber like you doesn't mean I can't sense things. You've been picking fights deliberately. You've been on my back and I've had just about enough of it. I can't relax in the house any more. Between your mother and you——'

'My mother has nothing to do with it.'

'That's what you think. Both of you hover over me like——'

'Not *you*, Jay. No one can get near you. The untouchable.

The unapproachable. You're so goddam cold. Why don't you send out invitations the nights you feel like talking?'

'You haven't lost your sarcasm, have you?'

'No. I haven't. But you sure as hell have lost any bit of tenderness you ever had. And believe me, that wasn't much.'

'So that's it!'

He pulled the car off the road.

'What?'

'This whole damn thing. You're mad because I'm not showering you with attention. Do you realize we have no privacy?'

'Now don't bring my mother into this again. Anyway, you couldn't shower attention if your life depended on it.'

'No. Of course not. I'm hard and cruel and unfeeling.'

'You're damn right.'

'Did it ever penetrate your thick skull that I may have problems, too? The residency? Worrying about you and Gary? And other things?'

'So talk about it! Tell me those things! I want to talk to you. But you're always in "yenem velt". You never ask me how I am today. You never smile or put your hand on my shoulder. Oh, yeah, you were sorry for me when I went to the hospital. But *I* went—you didn't. The bottom dropped out of *my* life, not yours. I'm trying. I'm really trying to get myself together again. But you don't help me. You never encourage——'

'That's a lie.'

'Is it? IS IT?' I was shouting now. 'You know something? I knew from the first days we met that you weren't tender or loving. Really loving. The way other men are. But I wouldn't admit it to myself. I'd excuse you in my mind. Oh, he's just reserved. That's why he doesn't squeeze my hand when we're visiting friends. Even if we are engaged. Oh, he just forgot to hold the door open for me and he just forgot to help me on with my coat and he just forgot a million other things a woman wants a man to remember. Look, Jay . . .' I spoke through gritted teeth, the words pouring out like water loosed from a dam. 'I know I'm not feminine and clinging and passive. I've talked to the doctor about that. It's part of my trouble. But you never helped me. You never made me feel like a woman.

Protected and petted. Even just a little. I've been afraid of you. Afraid to ask little favours. To help me with the dishes. Or take out the garbage. Or pick up a loaf of bread on the way home. So damn afraid you'd turn me down.'

'What did you want me to do? Read your mind? Did I ever refuse you when you asked me?'

'The way you did it. No enthusiasm. As though I were imposing.'

'What should I do? Jump for joy when I'm taking out the garbage?'

'You're just as sarcastic as I am.'

'You pick one or two things and blow them up so you can paint a nice black picture of me. What do you want of me, Judy? Really want?'

'A million dollars. Two mink coats. Jewels up to the elbows.'

'Is that your answer?'

'Don't be stupid. All I want is for you to be warmer. Have more feeling. Be more considerate. Is that so terrible?'

'Look. I'm no different now than I was six years ago when we were married. It's just not in me to be demonstrative or fawn over you. I can't help it. I'm not the hovering kind. But that business about not doing things for you is a damned lie.'

A muscle twitched in his neck.

'The trouble with you is you've always wanted more than I could ever give. You'll never be satisfied. Never. No matter what I do. You're like a child. You want constant attention. And I'm not going to fall into a trap like that.'

'Oh, yes. Sure. A trap. I ask you to be more loving and you call it a trap. What are you afraid of? Of being soft? Of being thoughtful? Kind? Great big strong man mustn't have a heart. Mustn't——'

'So get another man! Find someone who can cater to your abnormal demands and let you have a career and agree to no children.'

'My demands are *not* abnormal.'

'For me they are. Find someone who can satisfy them.'

My eyes swept his eyes and sudden fear clutched. 'I don't want someone else.'

'Then what *do* you want? Your father? I'm not like your

father. I never will be. And another thing. You're jealous of me. For being a man and having a career and not having to stay home and raise a family and be a woman. I don't hate you the way you do me. I'm sorry for you. And nobody can help you but yourself and the doctor. But mostly yourself.'

He turned the key in the starter. I wanted to say something. But the flood of rage was gone. I sat in silence.

'Before we go home,' he said, 'I want to tell you something. I'm definitely not reapplying to the University. I realize now you're not well enough. I'll look for a residency in Philly.'

The car rolled along the shoulder and bumped out on the highway.

'And no matter what you think, I want you to get well.'

Tuesday, April 3

It was almost like the first appointment, watching the hands of the office clock circle minutes into hours, with anxiety building until every muscle throbbed and every nerve grew taut. But this time the tension was rooted not in desperation, but impatience. I felt as though my skin would burst in the effort to contain my emotions.

I was twenty minutes early. I spent the time at the window of his waiting-room. I watched the clouds scud through the sky, the smoke plumes from chimneys torn by the wind, and the snail-like movements of the city below. I was trying to compose myself. But it didn't help. It never had. I could not break a mood or fear by concentrating on the world round me. Contemplation of externals seemed to accentuate the pain. I was a small, tight ball, a thing in a shell too hard to crack. The warmth of the sun, a bird call, a shaft of moonlight, laughter in the street . . . no sight or sound was strong enough to break me open and bring me peace.

The door opened behind me and I spun round to greet him.

'You don't know how I've waited to see you.'

'Why?'

'Something happened this week-end. I . . . I had it out with Jay. Do you remember, you told me to go home and think about my feelings towards him? Why I'm so afraid of him?'

'Yes. I remember.'

'A nice, quiet meditation. That's what I planned. And I'd come back here with brilliant discoveries and everything would be cleaned up.'

'Is that what you expected?'

'No. Not really. But I thought I'd have a chance to think and Look. We had a terrible fight and I'm all mixed up again——'

He spread open his hands. 'Do you want to start at the beginning?'

'Sunday we went for a ride. He called me sweetie and I blew up. I told him he was a hypocrite. After all the quarrels we've had he tries to sweet-talk me. And then everything mushroomed. We yelled at each other.' I rubbed my fingers across my forehead and stared at the floor. 'I didn't know I could feel such hate. When you're supposed to love somebody it's scary. I know about love and hate being together . . . you told me all that. But it's different talking about it and feeling it. Hearing yourself. Like dirty words. You understand?'

'Yes.'

'Well, that was just the preliminary bout. Then we got into the main event. I told him how cold he is, how hard, no feeling. I dug up things from the past to show him up . . . I mean, to prove my point. And he tells me I'd never be satisfied, no matter what he did for me. Well, that's a lie, Doctor Borman, that's a damn lie! If you could have heard him. He thinks my wish for attention is a trap. I don't want to trap him. I just want him to love me more. To show it. Is that a crime? Is it? *Is* it?

' "I can't satisfy you", he said. "Get someone who can. Go find your father." That's what he told me. What a lousy thing to say! He doesn't know how hard I'm trying to forget my father. I mean, work out my feelings. Why is he so goddam mean to me? He's worried, he tells me. About the future. Well, I'm worried too. What the hell does he think I do here twice a week . . . play gin rummy? If he'd only open up a little . . . talk to me. He's like stone. So cold . . . so hard. I can't move him.'

I blinked. The image of Jay's face was floating in the room. I saw his mouth with the lips tight and drawn.

My teeth clamped shut and a strange voice—was it mine?—growled up from my throat, hissing and vicious with an animal sound.   :

'I'd like to hit him . . . hard . . . and hit him and hit him . . .' My fingers clawed the chair arms and my eyes squeezed shut. '. . . and just keep hitting until I knock him down and break him open and spread him in pieces . . . tiny broken pieces . . . omigod!' My hands spread open on my lap and tears fell on my fingers. My glasses slid down the bridge of my nose. I reached up and pulled them off.

His shoes, his socks, his trouser cuffs. That's all I can see. Can't lift my head. Want to sit here and cry. Just cry. Then sleep. Long sleep. So tired.

'Doctor Borman, could I lie on the couch?' The voice still didn't sound like my own. It was so flat and expressionless.

'Do you want to?'

'I'd like to try it.' I forced my head up. Without my glasses his face was blurry. I coughed, rubbed my knuckles in my eyes, and reached for a tissue in my skirt pocket. I stood up. 'I don't guarantee. I mean, this is the first time. I mean, it's awkward. This business of lying down in the afternoon.'

I was by the couch now. I reached out and touched the leather.

It was cool. A nervous giggle bubbled.

'Doctor Borman, if a film producer stuck his head through that door now and yelled, "We're shooting a comedy. We need a lady who'll run up and down the hall in her bra and panties. We'll pay you twenty-five dollars", you know, I'd do it. Without thinking about it. But this . . . getting down on the couch. I'm embarrassed.'

'Would you rather try it some other time?'

'No. I'll do it now.'

I sat down and pressed my palms against the leather. Then I tucked my skirt round my legs and swung them up, and lay back on the pillow.

He got up immediately and sat in the chair I had been using. A lever clicked and the chair tilted backward.

It moves. Didn't know that. Reclining chair. Can't see him. Why didn't he tell me he lies down too? Don't like that at all. His feet . . .

sticking up . . . can see them . . . silly . . . my skin is crawling . . .
feel cold . . . and open . . . all exposed . . . dangerous . . . ripe for . . .
what? . . . death? . . . knife in the chest? . . . a stick . . . a thrust . . .

'Are you comfortable?'

'No.'

Want to get up. Can't. He's lying down. I'll be standing . . . on
top . . . bigger than he is . . . can't embarrass him, too.

'Try to relax.'

'It's hard enough to relax in my own bed. It's so strange here.
(*Why did I do this? I was so tired. Now I'm quivering. Couldn't sleep*
if he paid me . . . pay to sleep . . . oh God, what's with me . . . all
these sex thoughts . . .) Why do you lie down, too?'

'I find it's more relaxing to the patient.'

'Not for me.' I stifled another urge to stand up. 'I'd rather
look at you.'

'Why?'

'Don't laugh. But when I can't see you I don't know if
you're listening to me. Maybe you'll take a nap or file your
nails. . . . Oh, I heard a funny joke recently. There were two
psychiatrists riding in a lift at the end of the day. The younger
one says, "Fred, you've been practising for twenty years. How
do you stand it? Day in, day out, listening to other people's
troubles?" The older man looked at him and shrugged, "Who
listens?" There! You see? I told a joke and I can't tell whether
you smiled or not.'

'Is it important that I smile at you?'

'Yes, when I say something funny. And I like to look at
people when I talk. And I want them to look at me. That's
what makes me so angry with Jay. He . . . why did I say such
terrible things before?'

I squirmed and picked at my skirt.

'Did you think they were terrible?'

'My God! Didn't you?'

'No.'

Nothing is wrong here. Or right. No black or white. Curses or
kisses. Makes no difference to him. No lines drawn between foul words
or pure. No condoning. No condemning.

'But the words I used. The hate. For a minute there I didn't
know myself. Doesn't anything surprise you? I mean, when

somebody talks about the husband or mother as though they want to kill them?'

'I don't think you want to hurt them physically.'

'Them? What do you mean, them?'

'You mentioned your husband and your mother.'

'I did? Well, I meant anyone close. Father. Mother . . . Sister. The family. People you're supposed to love.'

'I understand. But you did mention your mother.'

'It was an accident. Her name just popped into my mind.'

'But isn't it interesting that you think of your mother in relation to your husband?'

His voice. Like a snake. Coiling at the back of my head. Squeezing my brains. What does he want from me?

'What's interesting about it?'

'Suppose you tell me.'

I giggled. 'I don't get you. I told you it was an accident. Don't you believe me?'

'I think you're avoiding something important.'

'You . . . you're trying to get me to admit something. I don't know what the hell it is, but I'm scared. I want a cigarette. Can I get up a minute?'

I sat up and reached for my purse on the end table. I kept my eyes down and away from him. When I lay down again, I drew deeply on the cigarette and exhaled. The smoke spiralled up and spread like a fog along the low ceiling, as if it were a trapped thing, looking for a way out.

'What frightens you?'

'The way you connect her with Jay. And those things I said about him. Wanting to smash and hit and tear apart. Is . . . is that how I feel about my mother?'

'What do you think?'

Why don't YOU know? You stupid doctor with your hot potato questions!

'All right. All right. For the sake of argument. So it wasn't an accident. So I want to tear her apart, too. But she's so different from Jay.'

'In what way?'

'A million ways. She talks. She talks all the time. About everything on her mind. Like me. Verbalizes all her fears.

Always asking questions. And she worries about everybody. Me. The baby. My father. Harold. Everybody.'

'Anything else?'

'Look. She's my mother.' I wanted to get up and face him and talk to his eyes instead of the ceiling. 'She's sixty years old. Jay is my husband. I just don't get the connection.'

'I see. All right. Suppose we stop here for today.'

His chair squealed and he was standing next to me, his trouser leg brushing my shoulder. I bolted upright, fixed my eyes on his belt buckle, and mumbled, 'This Friday, right?'

'Yes.'

'G'bye, Doctor Borman.'

'Good-bye, Judith.'

I was by the door when the words tumbled.

'This couch business. I . . . I don't know. It's upsetting. I'm more tired now than before. Just tired from laying.'

I closed the door and slammed my fist on my thigh.

You had to say something? 'Tired from laying.' Great exit line. Lay. That sex-word. I hate it. He must be laughing his head off. Next time I'll sit or stand or crawl up the wall but I won't get down on that goddam couch!

Thursday, April 5

Wonder if she senses it. The way I watch her, and listen while she talks. It's as though I've split into two parts. One part daughter, one part spy. She cuddles the baby and I stand across the room and scrutinize her face. She talks with Daddy and I hang on each word. She laughs. She frowns. She sits. She walks. And I watch and stare. Looking for evidence. Proof of her guilt. There has to be guilt somewhere. If I want to hurt her, she must have hurt me first. But when? And where? And why? She's Mother. My mother. I love her. I feel like a dirty sneak.

Friday, April 6

'Doctor Borman, do you mind if I don't go on the couch today?'

'No. Of course not. I told you to do whatever makes you feel more comfortable.'

'I want to tell you something. Lying down like that, it has a lot of sexual meaning. It's not relaxing. And I've got enough to worry about as it is. I'd rather sit up. All right?'

He smiled and nodded. 'All right. How are you doing?'

'I feel like a member of the secret police. At work I think about my mother. At home I watch her. Every move she makes. And I still don't see the relation between her and Jay. But you're the doctor. You must know what you're talking about. (*Wonder if that little dig hurt him? Want to hurt him. Putting me through this hellish maze.*) Can't you tell me? I've tried. Really, I've tried. You've helped me before.'

'Tell you what?'

'Why I made that slip of the tongue. Lumping hate for Jay with her. (*Is it still a hate? The fire's died now. I can look at Jay now without the gorge rising in my throat. There's just a hollow inside. Cool and empty.*) I'm knocking myself out and I can't make head-way.'

He hunched forward and folded his hands with the long skinny thumbs wagging in the air.

'Judith, I don't want to interpret a situation as important as this before you're fully aware of it. This is the hard part of therapy. I can lead. I can steer. But I can't bridge the gap of your own perception before you're ready to accept it.'

'But I'm ready, I tell you! I believe you. Anything you tell me. I'll accept it.'

'Why?'

'Because I have to know. I can't get well if I don't know.'

'That may be true in one area but not in another. How are you doing with your son?'

'A little better. But every time my mother goes out, even for five minutes, I'm nervous.'

'But you're less nervous than, say, two months ago?'

'Oh, yes. And I seem . . . I think I'm beginning to feel something. There are times when I can hold him and look at him and see how beautiful he is without thinking of how many polo shirts he has or does he need another blanket. Not all the time. But sometimes.'

Shaft of sunlight in the dark. Streaming warmth. Flowing, formless, yet strong.

'And the feeling is good?'

'Very good.' My eyes misted.

'I told you it could come in time. And it will grow even more. But not from my lecturing you on how to feel love for your child.'

'I used to ask you how, how, how. So many times. Didn't I?'

'Now as for this feeling about Jay and your mother. Here again you want a formal explanation. You have to feel it through emotionally, not intellectually.'

'Well, what should I do?'

'Let's talk about it.'

'You mean I should do the talking, huh?' I smiled at him.

He nodded, pulled at his moustache, and leaned back.

I took an exaggerated breath.

'I hate my husband because he's cold and unfeeling. He doesn't talk enough or show enough affection and attention. I'm always trying to draw him out. He hides from me. I don't know what he's thinking and I hate secrets. The whole thing is aggravated by my being sick. But it's always been there. I used to think I liked it. That cool, calm, collected manner of his. I called him my tower of strength. After all the talk, talk, talk in my own family. My mother always asked questions. My father always hovered. If I had a pimple on my face he'd come over with a worried look. They were both so much on me that Jay's disinterest was a relief. At first. Then I started to resent it. He was too much on the other side. And I never had the guts to tell him how I felt. I was afraid of him. And I still am. I've always been afraid of people like him. When they're quiet I think I've done something wrong and I'm being punished with silence.'

The sound of my voice had changed. I was no longer reciting mechanically. I was dredging up the words with effort.

'I think that they don't love me any more. So I have to keep running after them like a dog. Force them to open up and talk. And I hate myself for running and I hate them for being like that in the first place.'

I stopped. He hadn't moved. His eyes were focused on a point above my head.

'Do you want me to go on?'

He dropped his eyes to the clock ticking behind my chair. 'Yes. Go on.'

'I don't know what else to say.'

He smiled. 'You've said quite a lot.'

'But is it important?'

'I think so.'

'I still don't see what this has to do with my mother. I told you she's just the opposite of Jay. She talks about everything she sees and does. She can go up the street for a loaf of bread and a million things happen. She meets a lady with a dog who looks like our dog did. She had to go back for a blanket for Gary. Did I know they're selling frankfurters ten cents a pound cheaper in the store round the corner? They didn't have rye bread in the bakery so she had to get white and was it all right? That's the way she is. Everything has to be verbalized. I know I talk a lot, too, but sometimes it gets on my nerves. Like the blanket for Gary. When she said he needed a blanket because it got windy I felt it was my fault. I didn't anticipate the wind and protect my son against it the way she does. One minute I think she's trying to show me up for my lack of concern and the next minute she sets me up as the powerful one who has to tell her it's all right, little mother, that you chose white bread instead of rye.

'She confuses me. I never know where I stand with her. And now I'm grown up. I act very independent. As though I'm free of her. But inside I want her to tell me that everything I do is right. Why is it so important to me that she likes the dress I buy or the way I clean the house or how I cook a meal? I make believe I don't care, but I do care, very much. I'm always watching her face. Waiting for the smile and the nod and the pat on the head. I'm twenty-nine years old but I feel like a child with her. She's still the judge and the jury. And I'm still afraid of her if I do something wrong. I've got this feeling that she must approve. Then I'm safe. If she doesn't agree, then I'm not one with her. Not close. It's safe to be close with her. She may be nervous, but she's strong inside. She never complains of being tired. She's always the last to go to bed and the first up in the morning. She sleeps on a second-hand sofa bed that's hard as a rock and she says she likes it. In the coldest weather she goes out with her coat open at the neck and without a scarf. A scarf's too soft and tickles her neck, she says. She doesn't like make-up or perfume or dressy clothes or frilly things. She can't stand beauty parlours where people do personal things for you. She buys clothes only when she needs them—not when she wants them. I know. I'm like that too. So self-denying. But I'm not as strong as she is. I can't hold myself in the way she does. You know something? It's funny. I said she was a big talker. But it's always about the things round her. Not inside her. I know her face as I do my own but I can't really tell when she's happy or sad. She has no moods. If she does, I can't see them.

'Oh, when I was young it was different. I was a kid. She'd yell and hit me if I did something wrong. I could see she was angry. But I'm grown now. She doesn't punish me any more. We sit and talk together like people. Now I know this sounds screwy, but I don't really know my own mother. She hides from me. She says it'll be so nice when I'm well and she'll come to visit and it's wonderful that I'm living nearer to New York now and how good it is for families to be close. Stuff like that. But she won't let me get close to her. I told you I have to get close. Funny. My father always cuddled me and I couldn't stand it. And she. I wanted love and I couldn't get it. Physical love, I mean. Touching. Holding. Tickling. Anything. She'd kiss me good night but it was mostly a routine. Even now when I bend over her I feel so strange and awkward. Sometimes I want to go over and hug her, deliberately. Pick up her hand and kiss it. I know she'll squirm. Why the hell does she hide from me? Why can't I reach her? She's like . . . well, that clock of yours. See? I can turn and watch the hands move. I can hear it ticking, but I don't know what's inside. . . . That's her. She moves and ticks and we all looked to her . . . just like a clock . . . to tell you what to do and when to do it. She's always there. She's always right. Always important. But she's all closed up.

'I wish I could break her . . . shake her up . . . until the springs pop and I could see what the hell she is inside!'

I looked at my hands. They were balled into fists, the nails cutting into the palms. I opened them slowly, watching the fingers quiver with tension. They looked like live and wriggling things. I grabbed the ends of the chair arms and eased back.

There's a voice in this room, puffing and panting. Is it mine? And my chest. It's pumping up and down. And I'm hot. Steaming hot.

'I bet you thought I'd never stop talking. Did I bore you?'

Dig, dig, dig.

'No. On the contrary. It was very interesting.'

I wiped my face.

'I feel like I've been in a schvitz. Well, what do you make of my gibberish?'

'Do you think it's gibberish?'

'No. I wouldn't have worked up a sweat like this if I thought it was nonsense.'

'So. What do you make of it?'

I smiled wryly.

'You still won't put the pieces together for me?'

The moustache twitched. 'No.'

I sighed. 'Well, you don't have to. I can see it now. Jay and my mother. Alike. I mean, alike in the way I see them. Feel about them. You know, if you make yourself talk . . . force yourself . . . try to put feelings into words . . . sooner or later everything comes out. It's funny. I started out more to please you than anything else. To prove how far apart they are. And it ended up so differently. I hate them both because I'm afraid of them. And fear breeds hate, doesn't it? Afraid because they have this armour, this shell. They're so hard to crack. Too high to bring down.'

'From where?'

'From where they are. High up. Above me. I'm down here, see, and they're way up there. And I can't pull them down. I want to. How I want to! See? I'm angry again. I want to get at them and I can't. I just can't. I feel so impotent. As though I were flesh and bone and they were stone.'

'Why must you pull them down?'

'Why? If I could get at them I could be their equal. No more fear or grovelling.'

'I see.'

'Do you? Really?'

'Yes. I'd like to go into this more at the next session. All right?'

'But I've told you everything I feel.'

He put up his hand. 'I know. Let's just wait until next time.'

I sighed and half-smiled. 'O.K.'

He should hang a sign in this office. 'To the Patient: Remember, Your Best Is None Too Good.' No matter how much I tell him he says there is more to work on. No matter how far I go he wants me to go farther. Doesn't this twisty road ever end?

Tuesday, April 10

Well, what the hell is he waiting for? It's time for my hour. My hour is right. He sure makes me work for his money. Well, I'm finished. I emptied myself for him last time. Now let him do the talking. All those other aspects, those ramifications, those little some-things I'm always overlooking. Let him tell me. Tired of playing cat and mouse. He could help but he won't. Wants me to do everything the hard way. Sweating out every damn step. Sometimes I think he's just too lazy to answer me. Bet he goes home at night and cackles to his wife, 'That pain-in-the-neck patient was in again today, dear. The real pest. She wheedles. She needles. She begs. It's rather pitiful. Oh, well, what's for supper, darling? Chipped psyches on toast?' . . . What's wrong with me today? Is it the weather? So beautiful. Too beautiful to huddle in that musty room working up a cramp in the neck and smoking my throat raw. That afternoon, last August, in the hospital, when they let us out on the lawn and I felt the sun on my legs and rubbed a blade of grass between my fingers. Like waking up. Or breaking out. In the world again. Feel like that today. Want to be outside. Let the sun warm my face. Breathe clean air. Between the office and here and home I'm hardly ever out. And she's always telling me, go sit in the park. Take a walk. I'll make Jay's supper. Get out a little bit. Do some shopping. Go ahead, darling. Poor Mama. Poor, poor Mama. I love you and hate you and need you and want to be free of you. You're too good for me, too bad for me, too much for me. You——

'Hello, Doctor Borman.'

'Hi. (*The half-smile, the quick nod of the head, the hand on the door. The ritual of recognition. Always dread this moment when he's a stranger to me. In two minutes we'll be closeted together and he'll be picking my brains again.*) How are things? All right? I can't see much of it from here but it looks like a real Spring day.'

18

'Yes. It's lovely. Funny you should mention the weather. It bothers me. Oh, not like before, when I was so sick. Then I couldn't bear the sun or rain or anything. It just seems like too nice a day for . . . this.' I flung out my hands to include him, and myself, and the room. He was silent.

'Oh, I guess there's no point in using the weather as an excuse. I might as well tell you. I didn't want to come today. I'm angry at you.'

'Why?'

No consternation in his eyes. He's not afraid when he angers others, is he?

'You make me work so damn hard. I was exhausted when I left here last week. More so than other times.'

'Why?'

'Maybe it was the things I talked about. I feel like a louse. I do a hatchet job on Mother and then go home and see her taking care of my baby and my house. Living with me. Sacrificing so much so I can get well. I could choke from the guilt.'

'You're angry with me because we talk about your mother?'

'No. That's not your fault. I know my feelings are very important. It's just . . .' My voice trailed off and then grew loud. 'I get so mad when I sweat bullets here, trying to dredge things up, and you tell me there's more . . . there's always more. Another angle, another point. You send me home incomplete. You never finish anything for me. And I try so hard to do what you ask.'

'You're not supposed to do what I ask. Do or say what you want to.'

'Hell! If I did that, I'd take my coat and go home. Right now. But I can't. I'd have to pay you for the time anyway. Doctor Borman, I feel crummy today. Cranky. Tired. I know I shouldn't, but——'

'But you should.' He smiled. 'I remember in one of our early sessions you mentioned how controlled you used to be. No depressed periods. No moods or swings. What did I tell you?'

'That it wasn't normal.'

'Exactly. This attitude of yours today, it's a healthy one. I was wondering when you would show some slackening.'

'What do you mean?'

'No one can maintain a constant desire to produce in therapy. There are bound to be days when you'd rather not be here. When you don't feel like barrelling ahead.'

'And days when I'm annoyed with you?'

'Yes. Definitely.'

'But why should I be angry?'

He pursed his lips. 'Perhaps I'm not giving you the praise you need for your efforts.'

I was silent, picking at my fingernails. Then I spoke without looking up.

'You're right. I wish you'd shake my hand at the end of each hour and say, "Good work, Judith. You're coming along fine. Making great strides. You've got the courage to face yourself. I know how hard you're trying and I appreciate it. You're a very co-operative, intelligent, perceptive patient." But you never say anything like that. I feel so flat. Unappreciated.'

Bitter tears were squeezing from the corners of my eyes. I started as I realized he was leaning towards me, his fingers curled over his knees.

'I appreciate your earnestness, Judith. And your desire to progress.'

I flushed. 'Do you? Do you really?'

'But why this great need to be a good patient? Why do you want to please me so much and earn compliments?'

He had resumed his usual position in the swivel chair with his legs crossed high and his hands folded in his lap.

'I can't answer that question', I said, my voice tinged with anger. 'I don't know.'

'Do you want to talk about this?'

'I don't care if we do or don't.'

'You know, sometimes anger is a healthy sign. (*Great. Suppose I lay on the floor now and screamed and banged my heels. You'd pronounce me cured, huh?*) Particularly when we can trace its roots.'

'Look,' I said, 'I'm mad because I finally pull out of you a thanks for trying and right away you ask me why I need the support.'

'Not support. Praise, rewards.'

'It's the same thing.'

'No, it's not.'

'All right. It's not. I told you I feel cranky this afternoon. I'm sorry.'

'There's nothing to be sorry about.'

'So I'm not sorry.' I folded my hands and then forced the palms back until the finger joints cracked. The rage subsided and I looked at him contritely. 'Sometimes I don't know where I get the nerve to talk to you like this. I'm the patient. You're the doctor.'

'Yes. That's true in a technical sense. But not emotionally. Judith, I think I represent more to you than just a doctor. That's what I had in mind when I spoke of tracing your anger to its source.'

In spite of myself, the quickening of curiosity returned. 'Can we talk about it now?'

'Yes. Of course.' And he waited for me.

'Where should I begin?'

'Tell me why you want my praise.'

'Because I need . . . I need . . . ' I threw up my hands and laughed nervously. 'I just need!'

'What?'

'Encouragement. It's good for me. It spurs me, you know?'

His pale eyes narrowed very slightly.

He doesn't believe me, and I don't either.

'If I praise and compliment you, how do you feel?' he asked.

'Warm. Happy. Almost like a puppy. If I had a tail I'd wag it! And I want to do something that will please you again.'

'Since I dispense the rewards, how would you class our relationship?'

'Worker and boss, I guess.' I looked at him quizzically and immediately thought of Mrs. Meredith at the hotel office. Her patrician face stonily composed . . . the cool and distant eyes, and the tight lips that rarely smiled. No matter how many bookings I closed she never complimented or praised. She accepted all my efforts as a matter of course. And I wanted to please her, to force her approval. It was a battle in which I was always the loser because she was the boss, the ruler.

And I remembered how I felt, in the kitchen, cooking for Jay.

'I hate bosses', I said. 'People with power. People above me. You can't be equals with them because they'll fire you or flunk you. Take away the things you need.'

'What things?'

'Your pay cheque. Or a passing grade. Or your pride. Anything that's important to you. Security.' I bobbed my head. 'That's it. Security.'

'Would love be included with this security?'

'From a boss? Of course not!' I giggled, thinking, *what's the matter with him? I'm not that sick! Love from a boss!*

'Suppose we think of bosses in a broader sense. As figures of authority.'

Instantly I realized the significance of his question. The mental picture of Mrs. Meredith faded. Instead I saw my mother and Jay and remembered my desperate pleadings of the last session: 'If I could only get to them . . . pull them down . . . so I could be their equal . . . no more fear or grovelling.'

His face and body seemed to disappear, as if he were plucked away by a giant hand. I was alone in a corner of somewhere where hammers were pounding on my head, crashing in a soundless fury of insight.

Mama Boss and Teacher Boss and Professor Boss and Sir Boss, Husband Boss, Doctor Boss, Neighbour Boss. Everybody Boss. Everybody Stand Above Me.

The hammers stopped. His face was there again. He was watching me quietly, almost as if he sensed my turmoil and was waiting for it to subside.

I swallowed hard and managed a weak smile.

'Hello, Boss man.'

The bushy eyebrows knitted slightly.

'I've just realized that everyone's connected . . . everyone's a boss to me . . . whether they really are or not. Some people build castles in the air. I build ogres and idols. With one hand. With the other, I try to destroy them. My favourite game is Pedestal, Pedestal, who's on the Pedestal? Right now you're on the top. I want you to be nice to me . . . accept me . . . love me, I guess. Make me forget you're the boss. That's what I've done with my mother, isn't it? And Jay. And everybody. When they hold back I hate them and I get more afraid and the whole things goes round like a circle. How do I break out of it? How?'

, 'By becoming aware of the situation, as you're doing now. These feelings you have about people are important, of course. But they don't jibe with reality. You said before that everyone appears like a boss to you, whether they are or not.'

'Yes.'

'I think that's the crux of the chain reaction.'

'So who triggered it, my mother?'

He hesitated for an instant. 'I'd say it was the relationship you established with her which extended outward.'

'Jay is a man. But I see my mother's image in him. Is that it?'

'I would say so.'

'And all the others? The same?'

'Yes.'

'Well, it fits.' I smiled bitterly.

'What does?'

'I've always felt that I'm a child in a world of giants. Everybody bigger and stronger and more powerful. How do I knock them down?'

'By growing up to them. The problem is in yourself. You have to change the way you handle your own feelings. In all kinds of situations.'

'Well, how do I do that? How?'

I sensed the familiar surge in my body, as if I had sprouted a million invisible angers, all of them clawing at him, trying to back him in a corner and squeeze him until the ready answers ran out.

'You have to get an understanding of yourself. Then change will come naturally, without force.'

The fingers squeezed harder.

'All right. All right. So I understand what's wrong. So I become aware until I'm blue in the face. Then what?'

I heard the whining insistence in my voice. My eyes scanned his face for signs of annoyance. There were none.

'I know you want a detailed plan of action, Judith. But this is typical of your problems. The compulsive need for definite answers so you won't feel like a ship without a rudder. But any answers I give will act like a sedative. They won't help you understand the general anxiety you have about life.'

The fingers clawed again, this time in silent anger.

'Is that all you can tell me, Doctor Borman?'

'Right now, yes. Let me check our next session.'

He leafed through the appointment book.

'This Friday. Two-thirty. Is that all right for you?'

'Yes.'

He closed the book and watched me as I gathered up my things. My hand was on the door when he spoke.

'Judith, could you tell me exactly how your feelings grew for Gary? The steps you took or the plan you followed?'

The question broke sharply in the quiet room. I turned and saw him smiling with a gentle humour in his eyes. I tried to blurt out a reply. 'You mean the love I . . . the way it came . . . the . . .'

There was no need to struggle for words. I shook my head helplessly and tried to return the knowingness of his smile. I couldn't say it, but I felt it, like a warm wind rushing through me, singing and sighing. Lack of action is not inaction. No one can predetermine change in the surge of our emotions. We are as deep rivers, swirling with cross currents. We ebb and flow whether we will it or not. As long as we are aware of our turbulences, and allow ourselves the patience of experience, painful or sweet, time will create for us new patterns of existence.

'Hello. Jay?'

'Hi. How are you?'

'O.K.'

'What's up?'

'Nothing. I just got home and I wanted to phone you. Say hello. It's a beautiful day, isn't it?'

He laughed. 'I wish I knew! I've been in the operating room all day.'

'It's real warm. Like Spring.' (*Like love, Jay. Like health. Like peace.*) 'You'll be home tonight?'

'Yes. But late. About eleven.'

'I wish we could talk.'

'About what?'

'The situation.'

'Oh.'

'It's getting better. Really better. I have a lot to tell you.

'I'm glad. Very glad. I want to hear about it.'

'I wish you were home now.'

'So do I. I'll see you tonight, sweetie.'

I smiled at the word, the familiar word, the spur to my happiness, my anger, my tears.

'Yes. G'bye.'

Three o'clock. Eight hours to wait until I can share with him this secret inside. What will I say? That I'm better? I said that on the phone. That today's session was like a key thrust in my hand? Or a window opened after so much struggling and pulling? That I think I've turned a corner and all these months of plodding have suddenly lost their separateness? It's all of this and more. So much more.

My love for you, peppered with a hate of my own devising. My hunger for you; absolute, tyrannical, uncompromising, as a child for its father. My image of you, sprung from sick and tortured roots. He gave me a light, to see you as you are, not as I have created and distorted you. And a light for Mother, for Dad, for Gary. A time-light for my world and my people.

How demanding I've been of each day and each hour. How insistently I've pressed him and myself and everyone round me. I've always been a hurry-up cook, haven't I? Dump the things in the pot, even the delicate subtle spices, turn the flame up high, and give a violent stir every five minutes. I've cooked this way and cleaned this way, and worked and loved and borne a child this way, thrashing about with a fervour and a fear. I'm tired. Not depressed. Just tired. I want to let the pot simmer for a while. It won't be easy. I've been boiling inside for so long.

Remember how annoyed I'd be to see you sitting quietly in a room, your hands behind your head, your eyes resting on nothing at all? I was jealous of you, Jay, because in those brief moments you were free. You could savour a sense of peace I never attained in all my hours of feverish activity. I've flung myself headlong through life, dragging the demons of hate and guilt and fear. Like a cat running down the street with cans tied to its tail.

Remember that little trilogy you repeated to me while I was in the hospital? I love you. And you will get well. And it will take time. How sweet they were and then, so bitter. And when we fought I used them to taunt and ridicule. But now I want that time. Today and a month from today and a year or more. No matter how long he thinks I need. And I'll lean on you and break away; I'll fight with you and cling again. I'll close up tight one day and prattle the next. I'm going to feel feelings and accept them. I'll work with him to know myself and then ease up to let time set the pace.

There are tears on my face. I'm letting them fall. They feel so good. Like rain putting out a fire.

I rested my head on my arm. The afternoon sun streamed through the window. Across the street a woman wheeled a baby carriage. Two older children trailed behind. I thought, the grandmother has my baby out today. But that's all right. I don't mind. No wrench of guilt now. No wailing that it should be me, and why isn't it me? I'll wait. I can wait. Waiting isn't shame. Because each new day brings a new strength and a new growth. Just living is growing, if the inside eyes are open.

I must keep them open. I've been sick and I'm still sick. No use kidding myself just because I feel so calm right now. But I'm *getting better.* He broke open the fester, the core of me, and the torment and the pain ran out. It hurt. It still does. Maybe it always will. And there'll be more bitter pain as I dig and probe. But I'm stronger now. I know the enemy. It's me. Not my husband or my mother or my baby or the everybody-else. If I can take it easy and watch with those inside eyes and listen with inner ears and bend with each day as a young tree does in a storm, I'll grow and come of age emotionally.

I flicked away a speck of dust settling on the glass top of the desk.

I should be busy now. Wipe off the windowsills, sweep the porch, fold some nappies, or rinse out my stockings. But I don't feel like it. Right now everything can wait. This moment of peace. Too sweet to sully. There's another pram going by. When it's warm the babies pop out like daisies in the streets. I hope mother brings Gary home soon. Want to look at him and hold him and feel love flowing out. A giving, not a getting. Wonder if the answer is as simple as that. Sounds pretty, but too pat. There has to be self-love, too. A pride in being me. And courage. And control. And insight and patience to tolerate the bad days. And exultation for the moments of triumph.

'Live through it', he said. He might as well have said, 'Live.' I will. I want to. I've made a beginning.

· Now there is no end.

HAROLD M. IMERMAN, A.B., M.D.,

and T. BLANCHARD DEWEY

Introduction by J. D. Flew, M.D., F.R.C.O.G.

Obstetrical and Gynaecological Surgeon
University College Hospital, London

What Women Want to Know

A noted gynaecologist's guide to the personal problems of women's health

Far beyond the general books on women's health or sex or marriage, this book tells the reader in simple, non-technical terms,
what she wants to know, or should know. It is a specialist's book,
covering specifically and thoroughly the female reproductive
system and the disorders that may affect it.

Every pertinent medical matter is covered, not only the common
ailments and periodic disturbances, but also the more serious
problems and ills. In addition, full attention is given to the
psychological and psychiatric factors and the neuroses peculiar
to women.

This comprehensive, informative volume covers the whole life
cycle of womanhood, from the beginning of menstruation to
beyond the menopause. It is for the girl of fourteen, for the
young lady approaching marriage, for brides, wives, mothers
and those who want to be mothers, women who are approaching the change of life and those who have passed it.

> 'This is a good book destined to portray important informa-
> tion to the lay public. The book is clearly written and is very
> practical, and, what is more, it is accurate. . . . Every
> pertinent medical matter is covered . . . in addition, full
> attention is given to the psychological and psychiatric factors
> and the neuroses peculiar to women.
>   There can be little doubt that this book will be of value to
> nurses and students for it is an excellent introduction to the
> varied and many problems of sex, health and marriage.'
>   —MEDICAL PRESS

Obtainable from all good bookshops and libraries

MARY BARD
The Doctor Wears Three Faces

Highlights, and sidelights, on the everyday life of a doctor's
wife. You will enjoy being present whilst she operates on the
medical profession. The result is most satisfying.

'. . . bubbling humour, deep understanding, and high-grade
intelligence.'—JOSEPH TAGGART in the *Star*.

'This is a delightful book, in which sturdy common sense and an
ether mask are made amusing.'—CYRIL RAY, *Sunday Chronicle*.

BETTY MACDONALD
The Plague and I

Life in a sanatorium. Betty has scored another hit! She has
again written a witty, vivacious and *funny* book where, from the
setting, one would expect quite the contrary.

'A gay best seller—from the world of the sick . . . the book she
has now written is, in the highest sense, high-spirited.'
—PETER QUENNELL in the *Daily Mail*

'. . . as fresh as a daisy and as diverting as Danny Kaye.'
—GEORGE MALCOLM THOMSON in the *Evening Standard*

VICTORIA WOLF
Brainstorm

This is the story of a woman doctor's fight to save her marriage,
and her husband's reason.

'One of those strangely compulsive works of fiction that grip
and hold from the most tenuous beginnings, is Victoria Wolf's
Brainstorm. It tells of a shipboard meeting by two unhappily
married people, their marriage and the subsequent efforts of
the woman to save the life and sanity of her new husband when
his son is reported missing in Korea.'
—GLASGOW EVENING CITIZEN

Obtainable from all good bookshops and libraries

HAROLD M. IMERMAN,
A.B., M.D. *and*
T. BLANCHARD DEWEY

What Women Want to Know

'This is a good book destined to portray important information to the lay public. This book is clearly written and is very practical, and, what is more, it is accurate . . . Every pertinent medical matter is covered . . . in addition, full attention is given to the psychological and psychiatric factors and the neuroses peculiar to women.

'There can be little doubt that this book will be of value to nurses and students for it is an excellent introduction to the varied and many problems of sex, health and marriage.' – MEDICAL PRESS   *18s.*

BOEN SWINNY, M.D.

Conquering Your Allergy

Here is a book that fills one of the most urgent needs in the world today. Everyone who must endure the racking and debilitating discomfort of allergic symptoms will profit by carefully reading this book. Dr. Swinny shows with unusual clarity and simplicity what allergy is and what to do about it. He explains in detail the things the allergic can do to help himself and the kinds of treatment the family doctor as well as the specialist in allergy can give. His book should prove tremendously helpful to all allergy sufferers everywhere.   *12s. 6d.*

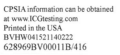